Table of Contents

INTRODUCTION

PURPOSE

Chemical warfare is not a popular topic, and most military health care providers do not willingly become familiar with it. This was painfully obvious during Operation Desert Shield/Desert Storm when it soon became apparent that many health care providers knew little about the effects of chemical agents or the medical defense against them. This ignorance was particularly striking in view of the seven-decade long history of modern chemical warfare and the well-publicized use of mustard and nerve agent during the Iran-Iraq War in the 1980s. The prevailing attitude of military health care providers was that chemical agents would be used only on Hmong, Afghans, Kurds, or similarly unprepared and unprotected groups of people. Further, many health care providers believed if chemical weapons were used the outcome would be disastrous, defense would be impossible, and the casualty rate and loss of life would be high.

Through education, however, medical professionals involved in Operation Desert Shield/Desert Storm learned that medical defenses were possible and effective, that chemical casualties could be saved and returned to duty, and that mortality could be minimized. Further, they realized that they might be the targets of chemical agents. More importantly, they rapidly learned that General Pershing's warning (written shortly after World War I) about chemical agents was still true: "...the effect is so deadly to the unprepared that we can never afford to neglect the question."

The purpose of this handbook is to provide medical personnel in the field a concise, pocket-sized reference source for the medical management of chemical casualties. It is not intended to be a definitive text on the management of chemical casualties.

HISTORY OF CHEMICAL WARFARE AND CURRENT THREAT

The use of chemical weapons dates from at least 423 B.C. when allies of Sparta in the Peloponnesian War took an Athenian-held fort by directing smoke from lighted coals, sulfur, and pitch through a hollowed-out beam into the fort. Other conflicts during the succeeding centuries saw the use of smoke and flame, and the Greeks, during the seventh century A.D., invented Greek fire, a combination probably of rosin, sulfur, pitch, naphtha, lime, and saltpeter. This floated on water and was particularly effective in naval operations. During the fifteenth and sixteenth centuries, Venice employed unspecified poisons in hollow explosive mortar shells and sent poison chests to its enemy to poison wells, crops, and animals.

The birth of modern inorganic chemistry during the late eighteenth and early nineteenth centuries and the flowering of organic chemistry in Germany during the late nineteenth and early twentieth centuries generated both a renewed interest in chemicals as military weapons and also a spirited debate concerning the ethics of chemical warfare. The British admiralty rejected as, "against the rules of warfare," an 1812 request to use burning, sulfur-laden ships as a prelude to marine landings in France. Forty-two years later, the British War Office similarly condemned Sir Lyon Playfair's proposal to use cyanide-filled shells to break the siege of Sebastopol during the Crimean War, arguing that to use cyanide was "inhumane and as bad as poisoning the enemy's water supply." (Sir Lyon retorted, "There's no sense to this objection. It is considered a legitimate mode of warfare to fill shells with molten metal that scatters upon the enemy and produces the most frightful modes of death. Why a poisonous vapor that would kill men without suffering is to be considered illegitimate is incomprehensible to me. However, no doubt in time chemistry will be used to lessen the sufferings of combatants.") Other nineteenth-century proposals that were never put into practice included the idea of using chlorine-filled shells against the Confederacy during the American Civil War and the suggestion of Napoleon III during the Franco-Prussian War that French bayonets be dipped into cyanide. The Brussels Convention of 1874 attempted to prohibit the use of poisons in war. Delegates to the Hague Conventions in 1899 and 1907 considered the morality of chemical warfare but were unable to draft more than a weak and vaguely worded resolution against the use of chemicals on the battlefield.

Against the background of this debate, World War I began. Early in the war, German units used the new, but as yet unreliable invention, the portable flamethrower; and France, where gendarmes had successfully employed riot-control agents for civilian crowd control, used small quantities of these agents in minor skirmishes against the Germans. Riot-control agents, although the first chemicals used on a modern battlefield, proved largely ineffective, and the search for more effective riot-control agents continued throughout the war.

It should have been no surprise that the first large-scale use of chemical agents during the war was by heavily industrialized Germany, with its impressive scientific base of theoretical and applied chemistry and its capacity for mass production of chemicals. German units released an estimated 150 tons of chlorine gas from some 6000 cylinders near Ypres, Belgium, during the afternoon of 15 April 1915. Although this attack caused probably no more than

800 deaths, it was psychologically devastating to the 15,000 Allied troops, who promptly retreated. The Germans, however, were unprepared to take advantage of this victory, and chlorine and its successors were doomed to play a tactical, rather than a strategic role, during the war.

Shortly thereafter, the British were ready to respond in kind with chlorine, and the chemical armamentarium of both sides expanded with the addition of phosgene and chloropicrin. These three agents damaged primarily the upper and lower airways, and both sides developed a variety of masks to prevent inhalation injury. Masks also had the potential to protect against cyanide, which the French and the British (but not the Germans) also fielded to a limited extent during the war.

However, on 12 July 1917, again near Ypres, Belgium, German artillery shells delivered a new kind of chemical agent, sulfur mustard, which in that attack alone caused 20,000 casualties and generated a series of new problems. Mustard, a relatively nonvolatile liquid, was persistent compared to the previously used agents, and thus not only the air that the soldier breathed, but also the objects that he touched, became potential weapons. It was effective at low doses. It affected not only the lungs, but also the eyes and the skin. Finally, the latent period of up to several hours with mustard meant there were no immediate clues to exposure as there had been with the earlier agents. Masks had to be augmented by hot, bulky, chemical protective clothing for soldiers and protection for their horses. The need for such a protective ensemble made fighting more difficult physically and psychologically. Diagnosis of mustard exposure was difficult, and mustard-exposed soldiers could easily overwhelm the medical system. Because the effects of mustard were delayed and progressive, most mustard casualties eventually presented for medical treatment. Although in most countries fewer than 5% of casualties from mustard who reached medical treatment stations died, mustard injuries were slow to heal and necessitated an average convalescent period of over six weeks.

Between World War I and World War II, debate on chemical warfare continued in the United States (U.S.) and in international forums. The wording of the 1925 Geneva Protocol, which all of the major powers except for the U.S. and Japan ratified, implied the prohibition of the first use (but not the possession) of chemical and biological weapons. The treaty preserved the right to use such weapons in retaliation for a chemical attack. Russia, which had suffered half a million chemical casualties during World War I, worked with Germany in chemical agent offensive and defensive programs from the late 1920s to the mid-1930s. In contrast, the U.S. Chemical Corps struggled to stay alive in the face of widespread sentiment against chemical warfare.

Evidence (not all of which is conclusive) suggests that the military use of chemical agents continued after the end of World War I. Following World War I, Great Britain allegedly used chemicals against the Russians and mustard against the Afghans north of the Khyber Pass, and Spain is said to have employed mustard shells and bombs against the Riff tribes of Morocco. During the next decade, the Soviet Union supposedly used lung irritants against tribesmen in Kurdistan; and Mussolini, who utilized tear gas during the war against Abyssinia in 1936 and 1937, also authorized massive aerial delivery of mustard (1) against Abyssinian tribesmen and (2) as an interdiction movement on Italian flanks. Immediately prior to World War II and during the early part of that war, Japan is supposed to have used chemical weapons against China.

In the late 1930s, a German industrial chemist, Dr. Gerhard Schrader, searching for more potent insecticides, synthesized tabun (GA), an extremely toxic organophosphate compound. Two years later, he synthesized sarin (GB), a similar but even more toxic compound. During World War II, Nazi Germany weaponized thousands of tons of these potent organophosphates that came to be called nerve agents. Why they were not used during the war is a matter of continuing discussion. Hitler, himself a mustard casualty during World War I, did not favor their use; neither did his senior staff who had fought on chemical battlefields during that war. Wrongly concluding from trends in Allied scientific publications on insecticides that the Allies had their own nerve agent program, German leaders may have been afraid of retaliation in kind to any Axis use of nerve agents. (President Roosevelt had in fact announced a no-first-use policy, but had promised instant retaliation for any Axis use of chemical agents.) Finally, during the later stages of the war, Germany lacked the air of superiority needed for effective delivery of chemical weapons. The well-organized German nerve agent program thus remained a complete secret until its discovery by the Allies during the closing days of the war.

With the possible exception of Japan during attacks on China, no nation during World War II used chemical agents on the battlefield, although Germany employed cyanide and perhaps other chemical agents in its concentration camps. However, over 600 military casualties and an unknown number of civilian casualties resulted from the 1943 German bombing in Bari Harbor, Italy, of the John Harvey, an American ship loaded with two thousand 100-pound mustard bombs. The 14% fatality rate was due in large part to systemic poisoning following ingestion of and skin exposure to mustard-contaminated water by sailors attempting to keep afloat in the harbor following the attack. Civilian casualties, on the other hand, suffered more from the inhalation of mustard-laden smoke.

The end of World War II did not stop the development, stockpiling, or use of chemical weapons. During the Yemen War of 1963 through 1967, Egypt in all probability used mustard bombs in support of South Yemen against royalist troops in North Yemen. The U.S., which used defoliants and riot-control agents in Vietnam and Laos, finally ratified the Geneva Protocol in 1975, but with the stated reservation that the treaty did not apply either to defoliants or riot-control agents. During the late 1970s and early 1980s, reports of the use of chemical weapons against the Cambodian refugees and against the Hmong tribesmen of central Laos surfaced, and the Soviet Union was accused of using chemical agents in Afghanistan.

Widely publicized reports of Iraqi use of chemical agents against Iran during the 1980s led to a United Nations investigation that confirmed the use of the vesicant mustard and the nerve agent GA. Later during the war, Iraq apparently also began to use the more volatile nerve agent GB, and Iran may have used chemical agents to a limited extent in an attempt to retaliate for Iraqi attacks. Press reports also implicated cyanide in the deaths of Kurds in the late 1980s.

Because of the confirmed Iraqi possession and use of chemical agents, preparations for the liberation of Kuwait by the United Nations coalition included extensive planning for defense against possible chemical attacks by Iraq. Even though this threat never materialized, United Nations inspection teams discovered nerve agents and mustard at Al Muthanna (about 80 km northwest of Baghdad) after the February 1991 cease fire. Other chemical stockpiles may yet exist in Iraq, and inspection efforts continue.

Other countries that have stockpiled chemical agents include countries of the former Soviet Union, Libya (the Rapta chemical plant, part of which may still be operational), and France. Over two dozen other nations may also have the capability to manufacture offensive chemical weapons. The development of chemical warfare programs in these countries is difficult to verify because the substances used in the production of chemical warfare agents are in many cases the same substances that are used to produce pesticides and other legitimate civilian products. The U.S.' stockpile consists almost entirely of nerve agents (GB and VX) and vesicants (primarily mustard [H, HD]). About 60% of this stockpile are in bulk storage containers, and 40% are stored in munitions, many of which are now obsolete. Since the

Congressional passage of a bill mandating the destruction of all U.S. chemical agents, one incinerator plant has gone into operation at Johnston Atoll, and other facilities are in the planning stages.

The chemical agents most likely to be used on a modern battlefield are the nerve agents and mustard; because of its alleged use by Iraq, cyanide may also pose a danger. Some intelligence analysts also consider the pulmonary intoxicants to be a credible threat.

TERMS

Chemical agents, like all other substances, may exist as solids, liquids, or gases, depending on temperature and pressure. Except for riot-control agents, which are solids at usually encountered temperatures and pressures, chemical agents in munitions are liquids. Following detonation of the munitions container, the agent is primarily dispersed as liquid or as an <u>aerosol</u>, defined as a collection of very small solid particles or liquid droplets suspended in a gas (in this case, the explosive gases and the atmosphere). Thus, "tear gas," a riot-control agent, is not really a gas at all, but rather an aerosolized solid. Likewise, mustard "gas" and nerve "gas" do not become true gases, even when hot enough to boil water (212°F at sea level).

Certain chemical agents such as hydrogen cyanide, chlorine, and phosgene may be gases when encountered during warm months of the year at sea level. The nerve agents and mustard are liquids under these conditions, but they are to a certain extent volatile; that is, they volatilize or evaporate, just as water or gasoline does, to form an often invisible vapor. A vapor is the gaseous form of a substance at a temperature lower than the boiling point of that substance at a given pressure. Liquid water, for example, becomes a gas when heated to its boiling point at a given pressure, but below that temperature, it slowly evaporates to form water vapor, which is invisible. Visible water clouds (steam) are composed not of water vapor, but rather suspensions of minute water droplets, that is, aerosols.

The tendency of a chemical agent to evaporate depends not only on its chemical composition and on the temperature and air pressure, but also on such variables as wind velocity and the nature of the underlying surface with which the agent is in contact. Just as water evaporates less quickly than gasoline does, but more quickly than motor oil at a given temperature, pure mustard is less volatile than the nerve agent GB, but is more volatile than the nerve agent VX. However, all of these agents evaporate more readily when the temperature rises, when a strong wind is blowing, or when they are resting on glass rather than on, for example, porous fabric.

Volatility is thus inversely related to **persistence**, because the more volatile a substance is, the more quickly it evaporates and the less it tends to stay or persist as a liquid and contaminate terrain and materiel. The liquid hazard of a persistent agent is generally more significant than the danger created by the small amounts of vapor that it may generate. The converse is true of nonpersistent agents, which may pose a serious vapor hazard, but which also evaporate quickly enough not to create a liquid hazard for an extended time. The arbitrary but generally accepted division between persistent and nonpersistent agents is 24 hours, meaning that a persistent agent will by definition constitute a liquid hazard and contaminate surfaces for 24 hours or longer. Such agents (mustard and VX) are thus suitable for contaminating and denying terrain and materiel to the enemy. Nonpersistent agents such as GB and cyanide find tactical employment in the direct line of assault into enemy territory since they will have evaporated within a day and will no longer contaminate surfaces. These generalizations are obviously subject to the modifying factors of temperature, environmental factors such as wind, and surface characteristics.

Biological effects occur following exposure to chemical agents dispersed as solids, liquids, gases, aerosols, or vapor. Eye or skin injury may follow direct exposure to the suspended solid particles of aerosolized riot-control agents, and inhalation of these agents brings the aerosolized solid in contact with the epithelium of the respiratory tree. Nevertheless, systemic effects from exposure to riot-control agents are rare. Contact of the eyes, or more likely the skin, with liquid nerve or vesicant agents may produce local effects or lead to absorption and systemic effects. Liquid exposure is the most important hazard associated with persistent agents and necessitates the proper wearing of chemical protective clothing. At low temperatures, hydrogen cyanide (AC), cyanogen chloride (CK), and phosgene (CG) exist as liquids. However, because of their high volatility (low persistence), they seldom present a significant liquid hazard unless the area of exposure is large or evaporation is impeded by trapping of liquid agent in saturated, porous clothing. Penetration of shrapnel or clothing contaminated with liquid chemical agent of any type may also lead to intramuscular or intravenous exposure and subsequent systemic effects.

Chemical agents in the form of aerosolized liquid droplets, vapor, or gas may directly contact the eyes, skin, or (through inhalation) the respiratory tree. Local damage is possible at any of these sites, but systemic absorption through dry, intact skin is usually less important than with the other routes. Vapor or gas exposure to the eyes, and especially the respiratory tree, is the most important hazard associated with nonpersistent agents and necessitates the proper wearing of a mask that provides both ocular and inhalation protection.

Specialized terms refer to the amount of chemical agent encountered during an exposure. The ED_{50} (pronounced "ED50") and the ID_{50} denote the quantities (usually measured as the weight in µg, mg, or g) of liquid agent that will predictably cause effects (E) or incapacitation (I) in 50% of a given group. Similarly, the LD_{50} is the Lethal Dose or quantity (weight) of liquid agent that will kill 50% of a group. Note that the lower the LD_{50}, the less agent is required and thus the more potent is the agent. Because of differences in absorption, the ED_{50} and LD_{50} values for a given agent are site-specific; that is, the LD_{50} for mustard absorbed through dry, unabraded skin is much higher than the LD_{50} for mustard absorbed through the eye.

Comparison of the amounts of chemical agent encountered as aerosol, vapor, or gas requires use of the concentration-time product or Ct, which refers to the agent concentration (usually in mg/m^3) multiplied by the time (usually in minutes) of exposure. For example, exposure to a concentration of 4 mg/m^3 of soman (GD) vapor for ten minutes results in a Ct of 40 mg·min/m^3. Exposure to 8 mg/m^3 for five minutes results in the same Ct (40 mg·min/m^3). For almost any given agent (with the notable exception of cyanide, which will be discussed in a separate chapter), the Ct associated with a biological effect is relatively constant even though the concentration and time components may vary within certain limits (Haber's Law). That is, a 10-minute exposure to 4 mg/m^3 of soman causes the same effects as a 5-minute exposure to 8 mg/m^3 of the agent or to a one-minute exposure to 40 mg/m^3. The ECt_{50}, ICt_{50}, and LCt_{50} then correspond for vapor or gas exposures to the ED_{50}, ID_{50}, and LD_{50}, respectively, for liquid exposure and are likewise site-specific. However, the concentration-time product does not take into account variables such as respiratory rate and depth and is therefore not an exact measure of inhalation exposure.

CHEMICAL AGENTS

Six types of agents will be discussed in this handbook.

Lung-damaging (pulmonary) agents include the World War I agent phosgene. The remainder of these agents are hazards of conventional warfare rather than chemical weapons. They include perflurorisobutylene (PFIB), a product of Teflon® combustion (Teflon® lines many military vehicles), HC smoke (a smoke containing zinc), and oxides of nitrogen (from burning munitions).

Cyanide has an undeserved reputation as a good warfare agent. Its LCt_{50} is large, and exposures slightly below the lethal Ct cause few effects. Its high volatility means that effective concentrations are difficult to achieve on the battleground, and that even high concentrations cannot be maintained for more that a few minutes in the open air. However, at high concentrations, cyanide kills quickly. Potential agents are hydrocyanic acid (AC) and cyanogen chloride (CK).

Vesicants include mustard (sulfur mustard, H, HD), Lewisite (L), and phosgene oxime (CX). Vesicants are so named because of the vesicles (blisters) they cause on the skin; however, these agents also damage the eyes and airways by direct contact and have other effects.

Nerve agents inhibit the enzyme acetylcholinesterase and effects are the result of excess acetylcholine. Nerve agents to be discussed are GA (tabun), GB (sarin), GD (soman), GF, and VX.

Incapacitating agents to be discussed include BZ, a glycolate anticholinergic compound related to atropine, scopolamine, and hyoscyamine, and Agent 15, an alleged Iraqi incapacitating agent that is likely to be chemically either identical to BZ or closely related to it.

Riot-control agents have been used on the battlefield, although they are not considered major agents of threat today. However, the National Guard may encounter or employ them during civil disturbances. The major ones are CS, which is used by law enforcement officials and the military, and CN (Mace®), which is sold in devices for self-protection.

HANDBOOK ORGANIZATION

The next six chapters deal with medical management of casualties from each of the six major groups of chemical agents. Following the chapters is a brief description of procedures for casualty management in a contaminated area. This is followed by a discussion of the principles of decontamination and a chapter describing equipment needed for chemical agent detection, protection, and self-decontamination. The appendices contain procedures for decontamination of litter and ambulatory casualties. Also contained in the appendices are tables listing relevant physicochemical properties and estimated toxicity data for these chemical agents, a diagram of the contaminated receiving area at a field medical facility, a diagram of the Personnel Decontamination Station, and a table briefly describing the agents.

PULMONARY AGENTS
CG

SUMMARY

Signs and Symptoms: eye and airway irritation, dyspnea, chest tightness, and **delayed** pulmonary edema.

Detection: **odor** of newly mown hay or freshly cut grass or corn. Neither the M256A1 detector kit nor chemical-agent detector paper (M8 paper, M9 paper) is designed to identify phosgene, but the MINICAMS, Monitox Plus, Draeger tubes, Individual Chemical Agent Detector (ICAD), M18A2, M90, and M93A1 Fox will detect small concentrations of this gas.

Decontamination: **vapor** - fresh air; **liquid** - copious water irrigation.

Management: termination of exposure, ABCs of resuscitation, enforced rest and observation, oxygen with or without positive airway pressure for signs of respiratory distress, other supportive therapy as needed.

OVERVIEW

Inhalation of selected organohalides, oxides of nitrogen (NO_x), and other compounds can result in varying degrees of pulmonary edema, usually after a symptom-free period that varies in duration with the amount inhaled. Chemically induced, acute lung injury by these groups of agents involves a permeability defect in the blood-air barrier (the alveolar-capillary membrane); however, the precise mechanisms of toxicity remain an enigma. The U.S. produces over a billion pounds of phosgene (CG) per year for industrial uses; however, we do not stockpile this agent for military use.

Perfluoroisobutylene (PFIB) is a toxic pyrolysis product of tetrafluoroethylene polymers encountered in military materiel (e.g., Teflon®, found in the interior of many military vehicles). The oxides of nitrogen (NO_x) are components of blast weapons or may be toxic decomposition products. Smokes (e.g., HC) contain toxic compounds that cause the same effects as phosgene. The remainder of this chapter will deal solely with phosgene because it is the prototype of this class of agents; however, the principles of medical management of phosgene exposure also apply to casualties from compounds such as PFIB or NO_x.

HISTORY/MILITARY RELEVANCE

John Davy first synthesized phosgene in 1812. Subsequent development as a potential chemical warfare agent led to the first battlefield use of phosgene (in shells filled solely with phosgene) at Verdun in 1917 by Germany. Later, both sides in the conflict employed phosgene either alone or in mixed-substance shells, usually in combination with chlorine. Although military preparations for World War II included the manufacture and stockpiling of phosgene-filled munitions, phosgene was not used during that war, and the U.S. Armed Forces do not currently stockpile this agent.

PHYSICOCHEMICAL CHARACTERISTICS

Phosgene is transported as a liquid. Military dispersion during World War I followed the explosion of liquid filled shells with subsequent rapid vaporization and formation of a white cloud due to its slight solubility in an aqueous environment. It spontaneously converted to a colorless, low-lying gas four times as dense as air. Because of its relatively low boiling point (7.5°C), phosgene was often mixed with other substances. It has a characteristic odor of sweet, newly-mown hay.

DETECTION AND PROTECTION

The immediately-dangerous-to-life-and-health (IDLH) concentration of phosgene is 2.0 parts per million (ppm). The M256A1 kit, M272 water-testing kit, M8 paper, M9 paper, Chemical Agent Monitor (CAM), Automated Continuous Air Monitoring System (ACAMS), M8A1 automatic chemical-agent detector alarm, and Depot Area Air Monitoring System (DAAMS) are all incapable of detecting phosgene (CG); however, the following detectors have the capacity to detect it at the threshold limits given:

DETECTOR	CG
MINICAMS	50 ppbv
Monitox Plus	0.25 TWA
Draeger	0.02 - 0.6 ppm
ICAD	25.0 mg/m^3
M18A2	12.0 mg/m^3
M90	>50 ppm
M93A1 Fox	115 mg/m^3

Because the odor of phosgene may be faint or lost after accommodation, olfactory detection of the odor of newly mown hay is not a reliable indicator of phosgene exposure. The eye irritation, coughing, sneezing, hoarseness, and other central respiratory effects seen after exposure to high concentrations are also unreliable guides to phosgene exposure, especially at lower but still lethal concentrations when they may be transient or entirely absent.

The activated charcoal in the canister of the chemical protective mask adsorbs phosgene, and the mask affords full protection from this gas.

MECHANISM OF TOXICITY

The pulmonary agents are absorbed almost exclusively by inhalation. Because they are gases, they readily penetrate to the level of the respiratory bronchioles and the alveoli, that is, to the peripheral compartment of the respiratory tree. However, most of these agents are essentially consumed by reactions occurring at the alveolar-capillary membrane or more proximally in the respiratory tract and are not systemically distributed to a clinically significant extent.

TOXICITY

The odor threshold for phosgene is about 1.5 mg/m^3, and phosgene irritates mucous membranes at 4 mg/m^3. The LCt_{50} of phosgene is approximately 3200 $mg\text{-}min/m^3$, which is half the LCt_{50} (6,000 $mg\text{-}min/m^3$) of chlorine, the first gas used on a large scale in World War I. Since only half as much phosgene is required to kill half of an exposed group, phosgene is thus twice as potent as chlorine. That it is less potent than almost all of the subsequently developed chemical warfare agents should not lead to an underestimation of its danger; deaths have occurred after the inhalation of only a few breaths of high concentrations of phosgene. Perfluoroisobutylene is ten times more toxic than phosgene.

TOXICODYNAMICS (MECHANISM OF ACTION)

Chemicals that are highly reactive or highly soluble in aqueous solutions (or both) tend to act in the conducting, or central compartment, of the respiratory tract. Most of the pulmonary agents are relatively insoluble and nonreactive compared to centrally acting irritants such as ammonia and hydrochloric acid, which cause pronounced irritation of the epithelial cells lining the upper airway on inhalation. Additionally, at low concentrations, they are essentially consumed by deposition and reaction in the conducting airways before having the chance to reach the peripheral portion of the respiratory tract. Peripherally acting agents such as phosgene, oxides of nitrogen, and PFIB are still largely unreacted by the time they reach the alveoli and the alveolar-capillary membranes, where they then undergo acylation reactions and are essentially consumed at that site, causing the damage that may eventually lead to pulmonary edema (see the section on toxicodynamics). However, it should be emphasized that the distinction between centrally and peripherally acting agents is not a strict either/or dichotomy. Centrally acting irritants such as hydrochloric acid (and the chemical warfare vesicants sulfur mustard and Lewisite, to be discussed in a subsequent chapter) when administered in high enough concentrations will not be entirely used up by reactions in the nasopharynx, trachea, bronchi, and large to medium-sized bronchioles. Enough of these agents may remain to act peripherally to cause pulmonary edema. Similarly, high concentrations of peripherally acting agents can release enough hydrochloric acid to cause significant central airway irritation and epithelial damage. Moreover, agents such as chlorine are approximately midway between the two poles of this spectrum. Chlorine-exposed soldiers in World War I usually exhibited both central airway damage and pulmonary edema, even from moderate concentrations of the gas.

Phosgene is only slightly soluble in water and aqueous solutions; however, once dissolved, it rapidly hydrolyzes to form carbon dioxide and hydrochloric acid. The early onset ocular, nasopharyngeal, and central airway irritation from high concentrations of phosgene results from the release of hydrochloric acid during phosgene hydrolysis by water in the upper airways. However, the carbonyl group (C=O) of phosgene can undergo acylation reactions with amino (-NH_2), hydroxyl (-OH), and sulfhydryl (-SH) groups, and these reactions account for the major pathophysiological effects of phosgene. Acylation occurs at alveolar-capillary membranes and leads to leakage of fluid from those capillaries into the interstitial portions of the lung. This effect is from direct contact of phosgene with these membranes; phosgene exposure by other routes, e.g., intravenous administration, does not cause this damage.

Phosgene-induced leakage of fluid from capillaries into the pulmonary interstitium is normally opposed by lymphatic drainage from the parenchyma, but as the fluid leakage increases, normal drainage mechanisms become progressively overwhelmed. After an asymptomatic or latent period of 20 minutes to 24 hours or longer, fluid eventually reaches alveoli and peripheral airways, leading to increasingly severe dyspnea and clinically evident pulmonary edema.

CLINICAL EFFECTS

Phosgene produces pulmonary edema following a clinical latent period of variable length that depends primarily on the intensity of exposure (i.e., the Ct), but also partly on the physical activity of the exposed individual. After the latent period, the patient experiences worsening respiratory distress that at first is unaccompanied by objectively verifiable signs of pulmonary damage, but may progress relentlessly to pulmonary edema and death.

During the time preceding the appearance of shortness of breath, individuals exposed to particularly high concentrations of organohalides may report symptoms associated with mucous membrane irritation. Exposure to large quantities of phosgene may irritate moist mucous membranes, presumably because of the generation of hydrochloric acid from the hydrolysis of phosgene. Transient burning sensation in the eyes with lacrimation and chemical conjunctivitis may coexist with mild, early onset cough and a substernal ache with a sensation of pressure. Irritation of the larynx by very large concentrations of the agent may lead to sudden laryngeal spasm and death.

A clinical latent period during which the patient is asymptomatic may follow low Ct exposure or the transient irritation associated with substantial phosgene exposure. This asymptomatic period may persist up to 24 hours after organohalide inhalation. The duration of this latent period is shorter following high Cts and is shortened by physical exertion following exposure.

The most prominent symptom following the clinical latent period is dyspnea, perceived as shortness of breath, with or without chest tightness. These sensations reflect hypoxemia, increased ventilatory drive, and decreased lung compliance, all of which result from the accumulation of fluid in the pulmonary interstitium and peripheral airways. Fine crackles appear at the lung bases, but these may not be clearly audible unless auscultation is conducted after a forced expiration. Later, auscultation reveals coarse crackles and râles in all lung fields, and increasing quantities of thin, watery secretions are noted. The buildup of fluid in the lungs has two clinically pertinent effects. First, developing pulmonary edema interferes with oxygen delivery to alveolar capillaries and may lead to hypoxemia, and if a sufficient percentage of hemoglobin is unoxygenated, cyanosis will become apparent. Secondly, the sequestration of plasma-derived fluid (up to one liter per hour) in the lungs may lead to hypovolemia and hypotension, interfering with oxygen delivery to the brain, kidneys, and other crucial organs. Death results from respiratory failure, hypoxemia, hypovolemia, or a combination of these factors. Hypoxia and hypotension may progress particularly rapidly and suggest a poor prognosis. The development of symptoms and signs of pulmonary edema within four hours of exposure is an especially accurate indicator of a poor prognosis; in the absence of immediately available intensive medical support, such patients are at high risk of death. Complications include infection of damaged lungs and delayed deaths following such respiratory infections.

DIFFERENTIAL DIAGNOSIS

Phosgene is distinguished by its odor, its generalized mucous membrane irritation in high concentrations, dyspnea, and *pulmonary edema of delayed onset*.

Riot-control agents produce a burning sensation predominantly in the eyes and upper airways. This irritation is typically more intense than that caused by phosgene and is unaccompanied by the distinctive odor of phosgene.

Nerve agents induce the production of watery secretions as well as respiratory distress; however, their other characteristic effects distinguish nerve agent toxicity from organohalide inhalation injury.

The respiratory toxicity associated with vesicants is usually delayed but predominantly affects the central, rather than the peripheral airways. Vesicant inhalation severe enough to cause dyspnea typically causes signs of airway necrosis, often with pseudomembrane formation and partial or complete upper airway obstruction. Finally, pulmonary parenchymal damage following vesicant exposure usually manifests itself as hemorrhage rather than pulmonary edema.

LABORATORY FINDINGS

No commonly available laboratory tests exist for the specific identification or quantification of phosgene inhalation; however, an increase in the hematocrit may reflect the hemoconcentration induced by transudation of fluid into the pulmonary parenchyma. Arterial blood gases may show a low PaO_2 or $PaCO_2$, which are early, nonspecific warnings of increased interstitial fluid in the lung.

Peak expiratory flow rate may decrease early after a massive phosgene exposure. This nonspecific test helps to assess the degree of airway damage and the effect of bronchodilator therapy. Decreased lung compliance and carbon monoxide diffusing capacity are particularly sensitive indicators of interstitial fluid volume in the lung, but are complex tests for hospital use only.

Early findings on chest x-ray are hyperinflation, followed later by pulmonary edema without cardiovascular changes of redistribution or cardiomegaly. Ventilation profusion ratio (V/Q) scanning is very sensitive but is nonspecific and for hospital use only.

MEDICAL MANAGEMENT

Terminate exposure as a vital first measure. This may be accomplished by physically removing the casualty from the contaminated environment or by isolating him from surrounding contamination by supplying a properly fitting mask. Decontamination of liquid agent on clothing or skin terminates exposure from that source.

Execute the ABCs of resuscitation as required. Establishing an airway is especially crucial in a patient exhibiting hoarseness or stridor; such individuals may face impending laryngeal spasm and require intubation. Establishing a clear airway also aids in interpretation of auscultatory findings. Steps to minimize the work of breathing must be taken. Because of the always present danger of hypotension induced by pulmonary edema or positive airway pressure, accurate determination of the casualty's circulatory status is vital not just initially, but also at regularly repeated intervals and whenever indicated by the clinical situation.

Enforce rest. Even minimal physical exertion may shorten the clinical latent period and increase the severity of respiratory symptoms and signs in an organohalide casualty, and physical activity in a symptomatic patient may precipitate acute clinical deterioration and even death. Strict limitation of activity (i.e., forced bed rest) and litter evacuation are mandatory for patients suspected of having inhaled any of the edematogenic agents. This is true whether or not the patient has respiratory symptoms and whether or not objective evidence of pulmonary edema is present.

Prepare to *manage airway secretions and prevent/treat bronchospasm.* Unless superinfection is present, secretions present in the airways of phosgene casualties are usually copious and watery. They may serve as an index to the degree of pulmonary edema and do not require specific therapy apart from suctioning and drainage. Antibiotics should be reserved for those patients with an infectious process documented by sputum gram staining and culture. Bronchospasm may occur in individuals with reactive airways, and these patients should receive theophylline, or beta-adrenergic bronchodilators. Steroid therapy is also indicated for bronchospasm as long as parenteral administration is chosen over topical therapy, which may result in inadequate distribution to damaged airways.

Methylprednisolone, 700-1000 mg or its equivalent, may be given intravenously in divided doses during the first day and then tapered during the duration of the clinical illness. The increased susceptibility to bacterial infection during steroid therapy mandates careful surveillance of the patient. No human studies have shown any benefit from steroids. Thus, steroids are not recommended in individuals without evidence of overt or latent reactive airway disease.

Prevent/treat pulmonary edema. Positive airway pressure provides some control over the clinical complications of pulmonary edema. Early use of a positive pressure mask may be beneficial. Positive airway pressure may exacerbate hypotension by decreasing thoracic venous return, necessitating intravenous fluid administration and perhaps judicious use of the pneumatic anti-shock garment.

Prevent/treat hypoxia. Oxygen therapy is definitely indicated and may require supplemental positive airway pressure administered via one of several available devices for generating intermittent or continuous positive pressure. Intubation with or without ventilatory assistance may be required, and positive pressure may need to be applied during at least the end-expiratory phase of the ventilator cycle.

Prevent/treat hypotension. Sequestration of plasma-derived fluid in the lungs may cause hypotension that may be exacerbated by positive airway pressure. Urgent intravenous administration of either crystalloid or colloid (which in this situation appear equally effective) may need to be supplemented by the judicious application of the pneumatic anti-shock garment. The use of vasopressors is a temporary measure until fluids can be replaced.

TRIAGE

Patients seen within 12 hours of exposure. A patient with pulmonary edema only is classified ***immediate*** if intensive pulmonary care is immediately available. In general, a shorter latent period portends a more serious illness. A ***delayed*** patient is dyspneic without objective signs and should be observed closely and retriaged hourly. An asymptomatic patient with known exposure should be classified *minimal* and observed and retriaged every two hours. If this patient remains asymptomatic 24 hours after exposure, discharge the patient. If exposure is doubtful and the patient remains asymptomatic 12 hours following putative exposure, consider discharge. An ***expectant*** patient presents with pulmonary edema, cyanosis, *and* hypotension. A casualty who presents with these signs within six hours of exposure generally will not survive; a casualty with the onset of these signs six hours or longer after exposure may survive with immediate, intensive medical care.

Patients seen more than 12 hours after exposure. A patient with pulmonary edema is classified ***immediate*** provided he will receive intensive care within several hours. If cyanosis and hypotension are also present, triage the patient as *expectant*. A ***delayed*** patient is dyspneic and should be observed closely and retriaged every two hours. If the patient is recovering, discharge him 24 hours after exposure. An asymptomatic patient or patient with resolving dyspnea is classified ***minimal***. If the patient is asymptomatic 24 hours after exposure, discharge him. A patient with persistent hypotension despite intensive medical care is ***expectant***.

RETURN TO DUTY

If the patient had only eye or upper airway irritation and is asymptomatic with normal physical examination 12 hours later, he may be returned to duty. If the patient's original complaint was dyspnea only, yet physical examination, chest x-ray, and arterial blood gases are all normal at 24 hours, he may be returned to duty. If the patient presented initially with symptoms and an abnormal physical examination, chest x-ray, or arterial blood gas, he requires close supervision but can be returned to duty at 48 hours if physical examination, chest x-ray, and arterial blood gases are all normal at that time.

CYANIDE
AC, CK

SUMMARY

Signs and Symptoms: few. After exposure to high Ct, seizures, respiratory and cardiac arrest.

Detection: The **M256A1 detector ticket** detects hydrogen cyanide (AC) as vapor or gas in the air, and the M272 kit detects cyanide in water. The ICAD, M18A2, and M90 detectors also detect AC. The CAM, M8A1 automatic chemical agent alarm (ACAA), and M8 and M9 paper do not detect cyanide.

Decontamination: Skin decontamination is usually not necessary because the agents are highly volatile. Wet, contaminated clothing should be removed and the underlying skin decontaminated with water or other standard decontaminants.

Management: ***Antidote:*** intravenous (IV) sodium nitrite and sodium thiosulfate. ***Supportive:*** oxygen, correct acidosis.

OVERVIEW

Cyanide is a rapidly acting, lethal agent that is limited in its military usefulness by its high LCt_{50} and high volatility. Death occurs within six to eight minutes after inhalation of a high Ct. Sodium nitrite and sodium thiosulfate are effective antidotes.

HISTORY/MILITARY RELEVANCE

The French used about 4000 tons of cyanide in World War I without notable military success, possibly because the small one to two pound munitions used could not deliver the large amounts needed to cause biological effects. Other factors included the high volatility of cyanide (which quickly evaporated and dispersed) and its "all or nothing" biological activity, i.e., it caused few effects because the lethal Ct (in contrast to mustard, which causes eye damage at 1% of the lethal amount).

The U.S. maintained a small number of cyanide munitions during World War II. Japan allegedly used cyanide against China before and during World War II, and Iraq may have used cyanide against the Kurds in the 1980s.

Terms. The term cyanide refers to the anion CN^-, or to its acidic form, hydrocyanic acid (HCN).

Cyanogen (C_2N_2) is formed by the oxidation of cyanide ions; however, the term cyanogen has also come to refer to a substance that forms cyanide upon metabolism and produces the biological effects of free cyanide (the term cyanogen is from "cyano" and "gennan," Greek meaning "to produce"). A simple **cyanide** (HCN, NaCN) is a compound that dissociates to the cyanide anion (CN^-) and a cation (H^+, Na^+). A **nitrile** is an organic compound that contains cyanide. A **cyanogen** usually refers to a nitrile that liberates the cyanide anion during metabolism and produces the biological effects of the cyanide anion. Cyanogens may be simple (cyanogen chloride) or complex (sodium nitroprusside).

Cyanides are also called "blood agents," an antiquated term still used by many in the military. At the time of the introduction of cyanide in World War I, the other chemical agents in use caused mainly local effects. Riot-control agents injured the skin and mucous membranes from direct contact, and phosgene damaged the lungs after inhalation. In contrast, inhaled cyanide produces systemic effects and was thought to be carried in the blood; hence, the term "blood agent." The widespread distribution of absorbed nerve agents and vesicants via the blood invalidates this term as a specific designator for cyanide. Also, the use of "blood agent" also carries the connotation that the main site of action of cyanide is in the blood, whereas cyanide actually acts primarily outside the bloodstream.

Materials of interest as chemical agents are the cyanide **hydrogen cyanide (hydrocyanic acid, AC)** and the simple cyanogen, **cyanogen chloride (CK)**. Cyanogen bromide was used briefly in World War I but is of no present interest.

Sources other than military. The cyanide ion is ubiquitous in nearly all living organisms that tolerate and even require the ion in low concentrations. The fruits and seeds (especially pits) of many plants such as cherries, peaches, almonds, and lima beans contain cyanogens capable of releasing free cyanide following enzymatic degradation. The edible portion (the roots) of the cassava plant (widely used as a food staple in many parts of the world) is also cyanogenic. The combustion of any material containing carbon and nitrogen has the potential to form cyanide; some plastics (particularly acrylonitriles) predictably release clinically significant amounts when burned. Industrial concerns in the U.S. manufacture over 300,000 tons of hydrogen cyanide annually. Cyanides find widespread use in chemical syntheses, electroplating, mineral extraction, dyeing, printing, photography, and agriculture, and in the manufacture of paper, textiles, and plastics.

PHYSICOCHEMICAL CHARACTERISTICS

The cyanides exist as liquids in munitions but rapidly vaporize upon detonation of the munitions. The major threat is from the vapor. The liquid toxicity is approximately that of mustard (see toxicity, below).

The preferred way to deliver cyanide on the battlefield is by large munitions (bombs, large shells), because smaller weapons will not provide the concentrations needed for effects.

DETECTION AND PROTECTION

The immediately-dangerous-to-life-and-health (IDLH) concentration of hydrogen cyanide (AC) is 50.0 parts per million (ppm); that for cyanogen chloride (CK) is 0.6 mg/m^3. M8 paper, M9 paper, the CAM, ACAMS, M8A1 automatic chemical-agent detector alarm, and DAAMS are incapable of detecting cyanide either as AC or CK. However, the detectors in the following chart are capable of detecting AC and CK at the threshold limits given.

DETECTOR	AC (Hydrocyanic Acid)	CK (Cyanogen Chloride)
M256A1	7.0 mg/m^3	
M272 (in water)	20.0 mg/m^3	
MINICAMS		130 ppbv
Draeger		0.25 – 5 ppm
ICAD	250 mg/m^3	
M18A2	8.0 mg/m^3	
M90	30 mg/m^3	
M93A1 Fox		46 mg/m^3

Because the odor of cyanide may be faint or lost after accommodation, olfactory detection of the odor of bitter almonds is not a reliable indicator of cyanide exposure, even for those who possess the gene required to smell cyanide. The activated charcoal in the canister of the chemical protective mask adsorbs cyanide, and the mask affords full protection from this gas.

MECHANISM OF TOXICITY

Cyanide salts in solid form or in solution are readily absorbed from the gastrointestinal tract when ingested. Moreover, the lower the pH in the stomach, the more hydrogen cyanide is released as gas from ingested salts. Liquid cyanide and cyanide in solution can be absorbed even through intact skin, but this route of entry is usually not clinically significant. Parenteral absorption of liquid cyanide can also occur from wounds. Cyanide is readily absorbed through the eyes, but the most important route of entry in a battlefield or terrorist scenario would likely be by inhalation. Following absorption, cyanide is quickly and widely distributed to all organs and tissues of the body. Ingestion leads to particularly high levels in the liver when compared with inhalation exposure, but both routes lead to high concentrations in plasma and erythrocytes and in the heart, lungs, and brain.

An example of the ability of cyanide to react with metals in the body is its reaction with the cobalt in hydroxycobalamin (vitamin B_{12a}) to form cyanocobalamin (vitamin B_{12}). The reactions of cyanide with metals are reversible and exhibit concentration-dependent equilibria, but the reactions of cyanide with sulfur-containing compounds are catalyzed by the enzyme rhodanese (EC 2.8.I.1) and are essentially one-way and irreversible. The rate-limiting factor in the rhodanese-mediated reactions is usually the availability of sulfur donors in the body. These reactions can be accelerated therapeutically by providing a sulfane such as sodium thiosulfate. The reaction products, thiocyanates and sulfites, are significantly less toxic than cyanide itself and are eliminated in the urine. Cyanide also reacts with carbonyl and sulfhydryl groups (directly or via 3-MPST and other enzymes). However, the two most important kinds of reactions from the perspective of understanding the classical mechanism of action of cyanide and its response to specific antidotal therapy are the reactions with metals and the enzyme-catalyzed reactions with sulfur-containing compounds.

Cyanide is eliminated unchanged from the body in breath, sweat, and urine - as sodium thiocyanate in the urine, and as iminothiocarboxylic acid (ITCA) from reaction with sulfhydryl groups. High concentrations of cyanide in the body will also lead to measurable increases in urinary elimination of cyanocobalamin (vitamin B_{12}).

TOXICITY

Cyanide is the least toxic of the "lethal" chemical agents. The **LCt_{50}s** of **AC** and **CK** by inhalation have been estimated to be **2500-5000 mg-min/m^3** for **AC** and about **11,000 mg-min/m^3** for **CK**. **LD_{50}s** for hydrogen cyanide have been estimated to be 1.1 mg/kg for IV administration and 100 mg/kg after skin exposure. The **oral LD_{50}s** for sodium and potassium cyanide are about 100 and 200 mg/kg, respectively.

Cyanide is unique among military chemical agents because it is detoxified at a rate that is of practical importance, about 17 mcg/kg·min. As a result, the LCt_{50} is greater for a long exposure (e.g., 60 minutes) than for a short exposure (e.g., 2 minutes).

TOXICODYNAMICS (MECHANISM OF ACTION)

Cyanide has a high affinity for certain sulfur compounds (sulfanes, which contain two covalently bonded but unequally charged sulfur atoms) and for certain metallic complexes, particularly those containing cobalt and the trivalent form of iron (Fe^{3+}). The cyanide ion can rapidly combine with iron in cytochrome a_3 (a component of the cytochrome aa_3 or cytochrome oxidase complex in mitochondria) to inhibit this enzyme, thus preventing intracellular oxygen utilization. The cell then utilizes anaerobic metabolism, creating excess lactic acid and a metabolic acidosis. Cyanide also has a high affinity for the ferric iron in methemoglobin, and one therapeutic stratagem induces the formation of methemoglobin to which cyanide preferentially binds.

The small quantity of cyanide always present in human tissues is metabolized at the approximate rate of 17 mcg/kg·min, primarily by the hepatic enzyme rhodanese, which catalyzes the irreversible reaction of cyanide and a sulfane to produce thiocyanate, a relatively nontoxic compound excreted in the urine. (An elevated concentration of thiocyanate in either blood or urine is evidence of cyanide exposure.) The limiting factor under normal conditions is the availability of a sulfane as a substrate for rhodanese, and sulfur is administered therapeutically as sodium thiosulfate to accelerate this reaction. The lethal dose of cyanide is time dependent because of the ability of the body to detoxify small amounts of cyanide via the rhodanese-catalyzed reaction with sulfane. A given amount of cyanide absorbed slowly may cause no biological effects even though the same amount administered over a very short period of time may be lethal. In contract, the LCt_{50} of each of the other chemical agents, which are not metabolized to the same extent as is cyanide, is relatively constant over time. A lethal amount causes death whether administered within minutes or over several hours.

CLINICAL EFFECTS

The organs most susceptible to cyanide are the central nervous system (CNS) and the heart. Most clinical effects are of CNS origin and are nonspecific.

Approximately 15 seconds after inhalation of a high concentration of cyanide, there is a transient hyperpnea, followed within 15 to 30 seconds by the onset of convulsions. Respiratory activity stops two to three minutes later, and cardiac activity ceases several minutes later still, or approximately six to eight minutes after exposure.

The onset and progression of signs and symptoms after ingestion of cyanide or after inhalation of a lower concentration of vapor are slower. The first effects may not occur until several minutes after exposure, and the time course of these effects depends on the amount absorbed and the rate of absorption. The initial transient hyperpnea may be followed by feelings of anxiety or apprehension, agitation, vertigo, a feeling of weakness, nausea with or without vomiting, and muscular trembling. Later, consciousness is lost, respiration decreases in rate and depth, and convulsions, apnea, and cardiac dysrhythmias and standstill follow. Because this cascade of events is prolonged, diagnosis and successful treatment are possible.

The effects of cyanogen chloride include those described for hydrogen cyanide. Cyanogen chloride is also similar to the riot-control agents in causing irritation to the eyes, nose, and airways, as well as marked lacrimation, rhinorrhea, and bronchosecretions.

Physical Findings. Physical findings are few and nonspecific. The two that are said to be characteristic are in fact not always observed. The first is severe respiratory distress in an acyanotic individual. When seen, "cherry-red" skin suggests either circulating carboxyhemoglobin from carbon monoxide poisoning or high venous oxygen content from failure of extraction of oxygen by tissues poisoned by cyanide or hydrogen sulfide. However, cyanide victims may have normal appearing skin and may even be cyanotic, although cyanosis is not classically associated with cyanide poisoning.

Table. Cyanide (AC and CK)
Effects from Vapor Exposure

Moderate, from low concen-tration	Transient increase in rate and depth of breathing, dizziness, nausea, vomiting, headache.	These may progress to severe effects if exposure continues.	The time of onset of these effects depends on the concen-tration but is often within minutes after onset of exposure.
Severe, from high concen-tration	Transient increase in rate and depth of breathing - 15 seconds. Convulsions - 30 seconds. Cessation of respiration - 2 to 4 minutes. Cessation of heartbeat - 4 to 8 minutes.		

In addition to the preceding effects, CK causes intense irritation of the eyes, nose, and airways.

The second classic sign of cyanide poisoning is the odor of bitter almonds; however, approximately 50% of the population are genetically unable to detect the odor of cyanide.

The casualty may be diaphoretic with normal sized or large pupils. A declining blood pressure and tachycardia follow an initial hypertension and compensatory bradycardia. Terminal hypotension is accompanied by bradyrhythmias before asystole.

TIME COURSE OF EFFECTS

Effects begin 15 seconds following inhalation of a lethal Ct; death ensues in 6 to 8 minutes. The onset of effects following inhalation of lower Cts may be as early as minutes after the onset of exposure. After exposure is terminated by evacuation to fresh air or by masking, there is little danger of delayed onset of effects.

DIFFERENTIAL DIAGNOSIS

Battlefield inhalation exposure to either cyanide or a nerve agent may precipitate the sudden onset of loss of consciousness followed by convulsions and apnea. The nerve agent casualty has miosis (until shortly before death), copious oral and nasal secretions, and muscular fasciculations. The cyanide casualty has normal sized or dilated pupils, few secretions, and muscular twitching, but no fasciculations. In addition, the nerve agent casualty may be cyanotic, whereas the cyanide casualty usually is not.

LABORATORY FINDINGS

1. ***An elevated blood cyanide concentration.*** Mild effects may be apparent at concentrations of 0.5 to 1.0 mcg/ml, and concentrations of 2.5 mcg/ml and higher are associated with coma, convulsions, and death.

2. ***Acidosis.*** Metabolic acidosis with a high concentration of lactic acid (lactic acidosis) or a metabolic acidosis with an unusually high anion gap (if the means to measure lactic acid are not available) may be present. Because oxygen cannot be utilized, anaerobic metabolism with the production of lactic acid replaces aerobic metabolism. Lactic acidosis, however, may reflect other disease states and is not specific for cyanide poisoning.

3. ***Oxygen content of venous blood greater than normal.*** This also is a result of poisoning of the intramitochondrial respiratory chain and the resulting

failure of cells to extract oxygen from arterial blood. This finding is also not specific for cyanide poisoning.

MEDICAL MANAGEMENT

Management of cyanide poisoning begins with removal to fresh air. Dermal decontamination is unnecessary if exposure has been only to vapor, but wet clothing should be removed and the underlying skin should be washed either with soap and water or water alone if liquid on the skin is a possibility. Attention to the basics of intensive supportive care is critical and includes mechanical ventilation as needed, circulatory support with crystalloids and vasopressors, correction of metabolic acidosis with IV sodium bicarbonate, and seizure control with benzodiazepine administration. The fact that cyanide inhibits cellular utilization of oxygen would lead to the expectation that supplemental oxygen would not be of use in cyanide poisoning. However, in fact, administration of 100% oxygen has been found empirically to exert a beneficial effect and should be a part of general supportive care for every cyanide-poisoned patient.

Symptomatic patients, especially those with severe manifestations, may further benefit from specific antidotal therapy. This is provided in a two-step process. First, a methemoglobin-forming agent such as amyl nitrite (available in civilian antidote kits, but not in military kits, as crushable ampoules for inhalation) or sodium nitrite (for intravenous use) is administered, since the ferric ion (Fe^{3+}) in methemoglobin has an even higher affinity for cyanide than does cytochrome a_3. The equilibrium of this reaction causes dissociation of bound cyanide from cytochrome a_3 and frees the enzyme to help produce ATP again. The orthostatic hypotension produced by nitrite administration is not usually a concern in a severely intoxicated and prostrate cyanide casualty, but overproduction of methemoglobin may compromise oxygen-carrying capacity. Thus, nitrite is relatively contraindicated in, for example, smoke-inhalation victims. The initial adult dose, equivalent to one of the two sodium nitrite vials in the standard Pasadena (formerly Lilly) Cyanide Antidote Kit, is 10 ml. Pediatric nitrite dosing (in the case of a military response to a civilian terrorist incident) is dependent on body weight and hemoglobin concentration. The recommended pediatric dose, assuming a hemoglobin concentration of 12 g/dl, is 0.33 ml/kg of the standard 3% solution given slowly, IV, over 5 to 10 minutes.

The second step is provision of a sulfur donor, typically sodium thiosulfate, which is utilized as a substrate by rhodanese for its conversion of cyanide to thiocyanate. Sodium thiosulfate itself is efficacious, relatively benign, and also synergistic with oxygen administration and thus may be used without nitrites empirically in situations such as smoke inhalation with high carboxyhemoglobin levels. The initial adult dose, equivalent to one of the two large bottles in the Pasadena Kit, is 50 ml; the initial thiosulfate dose for pediatric patients is 1.65 ml/kg of the standard 25% solution, IV. Second treatments with each of the two antidotes may be given at up to half the original dose if needed.

It is important to realize that, although the combination of sodium nitrite and sodium thiosulfate may save victims exposed to 10 to 20 lethal doses of cyanide and are effective even after breathing has stopped, many patients will recover even without specific antidotal treatment if vigorous general supportive care is emphasized. Lack of availability of antidotes is therefore not a reason to consider even apneic cyanide casualties expectant. It is also important to realize that administration of antidotes, especially if not given slowly enough or if given in extremely large doses, is also associated with morbidity and even mortality. Antidotes should not be withheld in a patient in whom cyanide poisoning is suspected, but infusion rates should be slow and the drugs should be titrated to effect. Overdosage should be avoided.

Several alternative therapies and experimental antidotes are used in other NATO countries. Germany uses dimethylaminophenol (DMAP), a rapid methemoglobin former developed for intramuscular

(IM) use. However, muscle necrosis at the site of injection occurs, and only the IV route of administration is recommended.

Certain cobalt compounds directly chelate cyanide to reduce its toxicity. Because cobalt compounds do not depend upon the formation of methemoglobin, they may exert their antidotal activity more quickly than do methemoglobin-formers. Great Britain and France use cobalt edetate (Kelocyanor), but clear superiority to the methemoglobin formers has not been demonstrated, and cobalt toxicity is occasionally seen, particularly if the patient has only a mild exposure. The other cobalt compound sometimes used in France is hydroxycobalamin (vitamin B_{12a}), which complexes with cyanide on a molar basis. Clinical trials of this compound are underway in the U.S..

Ongoing research is examining whether slow methemoglobin formers can be used as pretreatment to induce clinically asymptomatic methemoglobinemia in troops at high risk for cyanide exposure.

TRIAGE

An **immediate** casualty is one who presents within minutes of inhalation exposure with convulsions or the recent onset of apnea, but with circulation intact. Immediate antidote administration will be lifesaving.

A **minimal** casualty is one who has inhaled less than a lethal amount and has mild effects. The antidotes may reduce his symptoms but are not lifesaving.

The **delayed** casualty is one recovering from mild effects or successful therapy. Generally, it will be hours before full recovery. Evacuation is not necessary but might be considered until full recovery takes place.

An **expectant** casualty is apneic with circulatory failure.

Generally, a casualty who has had inhalation exposure and survives long enough to reach medical care will need little treatment.

RETURN TO DUTY

Full recovery is usually relatively fast after cyanide intoxication. Those with mild to moderate effects from the agent can usually return to duty within hours, and those successfully treated after severe effects can return within a day.

VESICANTS
HD, H, L, CX

OVERVIEW

Sulfur mustard has posed a military threat since its introduction on the battlefield in World War I. Most of this chapter concerns this agent. Unless otherwise noted, the term "mustard" refers to sulfur mustard.

The nitrogen mustards (HN1, HN2, and HN3) were synthesized in the 1930s, but were not produced in large amounts for warfare. Mechlorethamine (HN2, Mustargen) became the prototypical cancer chemotherapeutic compound and remained the standard compound for this purpose for many years.

Lewisite (L) was synthesized during the late stages of World War I, but probably has not been used on a battlefield. The Lewisite antidote, British-Anti-Lewisite (BAL), finds medicinal use today as a heavy-metal chelator.

Although classified as a vesicant, phosgene oxime (CX) is a corrosive urticant that also has not seen battlefield use.

Lewisite and phosgene oxime pose only minor potential military threats and will be discussed briefly at the end of this chapter.

MUSTARD
HD, H

SUMMARY

Signs and Symptoms: asymptomatic latent period (hours). Erythema and blisters on the **skin**; irritation, conjunctivitis, corneal opacity, and damage in the **eyes**; mild upper respiratory signs to marked **airway** damage; also gastrointestinal (GI) effects and bone marrow stem cell suppression.

Detection: M256A1, M272 water testing kit, MINICAMS, the ICAD, M18A2, M21 remote sensing alarm, M90, M93A1 Fox, Bubbler, CAM, and DAAMS (but **NOT** the M8A1 automatic chemical agent alarm), M8 paper, or M9 paper.

Decontamination: 0.5% hypochlorite, M291 kit, and water in large amounts.

Management: Decontamination immediately after exposure is the only way to prevent damage. Supportive care of patients - there is no specific therapy.

OVERVIEW

Vesicant agents, specifically sulfur mustard (H, HD), have been major military threat agents since their introduction in World War I. They constitute both a vapor and a liquid threat to all exposed skin and mucous membranes. Mustard's effects are delayed, appearing hours after exposure. The organs most commonly affected are the skin (with erythema and vesicles), eyes (with mild conjunctivitis to severe eye damage), and airways (with mild irritation of the upper respiratory tract, to severe bronchiolar damage leading to necrosis and hemorrhage of the airway mucosa and musculature). Following exposure to large quantities of mustard, precursor cells of the bone marrow are damaged, leading to pancytopenia and increased susceptibility to infection. The GI tract may be damaged, and there are sometimes central nervous system signs. There is no specific antidote, and management is symptomatic therapy. Immediate decontamination is the only way to reduce damage.

HISTORY/MILITARY RELEVANCE

Sulfur mustard was first synthesized in the early 1800s and was first used on the battlefield during World War I by Germany in July 1917. Despite its introduction late in that conflict, mustard produced the most chemical casualties, although fewer than 5%

of the casualties who reached medical treatment facilities died. Italy allegedly used mustard in the 1930s against Abyssinia. Egypt apparently employed mustard in the 1960s against Yemen, and Iraq used mustard in the 1980s against Iran and the Kurds. Mustard is still considered a major threat agent of former Warsaw Pact countries and third world countries.

The U.S. manufactured mustard during World War I and World War II and maintains a stockpile that is currently undergoing destruction.

Nomenclature. Sulfur mustard manufactured by the Levinstein process contains up to 30% impurities (mostly sulfur) and is known as H. Mustard made by a distillation procedure is almost pure and is known as HD (distilled mustard). An early term for the German agent was HS (probably derived from the World War I slang term, Hun Stoffe).

PHYSICOCHEMICAL CHARACTERISTICS

Mustard is an oily liquid with a color ranging from light yellow to brown. Its odor is that of garlic, onion, or mustard (hence its name), but because of accommodation of the sense of smell, odor should not be relied on for detection. Under temperate conditions, mustard evaporates slowly and is primarily a liquid hazard, but its vapor hazard increases with increasing temperature. At 100°F or above, it is a definite vapor hazard. Mustard freezes at 57°F, and since a solid is difficult to disperse, mustard is often mixed with substances with a lower freezing point, e.g., Lewisite (the mixture is HL), or agent T, a closely related vesicant (the mixture is HT) so that the mixture will remain liquid at lower temperatures. The mixture HT also refers to mustard that has been thickened with small quantities of newer thickening agents.

DETECTION AND PROTECTION

The immediately-dangerous-to-life-and-health (IDLH) concentration of sulfur mustard (H) is 0.003 mg/m3. The M8A1 automatic chemical agent detector alarm is incapable of detecting mustard. However, liquid mustard turns M8 paper a ketchup red, and M9 paper will turn pink, red, reddish-brown, or purple when exposed to liquid nerve agents or vesicants, but does not specifically identify either the class of agent or the specific agent. The detectors in the following chart have the capacity to detect sulfur mustard (H) at the threshold limits given.

DETECTOR	H
M256A1	3.0 mg/min^3
M272 (in water)	2.0 mg/min^3
MINICAMS	0.00003 mg/min^3
ICAD	10.0 mg/min^3
M18A2	0.5 mg/min^3
M21	150 mg/min^3
M90	0.2 mg/min^3
M93A1 Fox	0.01 - 1 mcg/l
ACAMS	0.003 mg/min^3
Bubbler	0.003 mg/min^3
CAM	0.1 mg/min^3
DAAMS	0.003 mg/min^3

Because the odor of sulfur mustard may be faint or lost after accommodation, olfactory detection of the odor of mustard, garlic, onions, or horseradish is not a reliable indicator of mustard exposure. The activated charcoal in the canister of the chemical protective mask adsorbs mustard, as does the charcoal in the chemical protective overgarment. The butyl rubber in the chemical protective gloves and boots is impermeable to mustard. Proper wear of the chemical protective mask and the chemical protective ensemble affords full protection against sulfur mustard.

MECHANISM OF TOXICITY

Mustard vapor and liquid readily penetrate thin layers of most fabrics (but not the chemical protective ensemble) to reach underlying skin. Although mustard dissolves relatively slowly in aqueous solutions such as sweat, the lipophilicity of mustard guarantees effective absorption through even intact skin. Penetration is rapid (1 to 4 mcg/cm^2-min) and is enhanced by moisture, heat, and thin skin. This explains the otherwise baffling observation that World War I mustard burns involved the scrotum in 42% of cases, but the presumably more readily exposed hands in only 4% of cases. Ocular and respiratory routes of entry are also important, as is parenteral absorption in casualties with conventional wounds. Ingestion (enteral absorption) was an important route of entry for mustard in the sailors exposed outside Bari in World War II. Approximately 10% of the amount of mustard that begins to penetrate the skin will bind to the skin as "fixed" (reacted) mustard; the remaining 90% of the dose reaches the circulation and is systemically distributed as "free" (unreacted and hydrolyzed) mustard. Distribution to almost all organs and tissues including the kidneys, liver, intestines, and lungs occurs; although, because of dilutional effects and reactions of mustard in the bloodstream, clinical effects from systemic distribution are seen only at high doses. After IV administration, mustard disappears from the blood within seconds to minutes. Because of the rapid fixation of mustard to tissue, the fluid inside the blisters that eventually develop at the sites of skin contact contains no free mustard and does not pose a contamination hazard to health care providers. Mustard participates in a variety of biotransformative (metabolic) reactions in the body. Some of these reactions are catalyzed by enzymes, but most absorbed mustard reacts directly by forming covalent bonds (via alkylation) with DNA, RNA, proteins, components of cell membranes, and other macromolecules in the body. Mustard is eliminated primarily in the urine as by-products of alkylation.

TOXICITY

The LCt_{50} of sulfur mustard dispersed as a vapor is 1500 mg-min/m^3 in an unprotected group and 10,000 mg-min/m^3 in a group with respiratory protection. This demonstrates not only the importance of respiratory protection, but also the fact that sufficient concentrations of vapor and sufficient exposure times render mustard vapor lethal, even in masked individuals. The LD_{50} of liquid mustard on the skin is 100 mg/kg. Thus, administration of 7 g (about a teaspoon) of liquid mustard to each member of a group of individuals weighing 70 kg would be expected to cause the death of half of those exposed. Although 7 g of a liquid applied evenly to the surface of the skin may cover approximately 20 to 25% of the total body surface area (BSA), the correlation between BSA involvement and deaths from mustard in the field is poor. One plausible reason for this discrepancy is that using BSA figures by themselves ignore the inhalational component of mustard exposure. Another conceivable explanation is that measurement solely of affected BSA neglects factors such as the thickness of coverage, subsequent spread, contact time, and continued exposure. A 10 mcg droplet of sulfur mustard can produce a small vesicle on exposed skin.

TOXICODYNAMICS (MECHANISM OF ACTION)

Absorbed mustard must first dissolve in aqueous solution such as sweat or extracellular fluid. Although mustard molecules dissolve slowly in such solutions, once they dissolve they rapidly (within seconds to a minute or two) rearrange to form extremely reactive cyclic ethylene sulfonium ions that immediately bind to intracellular and extracellular enzymes, proteins, and other cellular components. Mustard has many biological actions, but the exact mechanism by which it produces tissue injury is not known. According to one prominent hypothesis, biological damage from mustard results from DNA alkylation and crosslinking in rapidly dividing cells, such as basal keratinocytes, mucosal epithelium, and bone marrow precursor cells. This leads to cellular death and inflammatory reaction, and, in the skin, protease digestion of anchoring filaments at the epidermal-dermal junction and the formation of blisters.

Mustard also possesses mild cholinergic activity, which may be responsible for effects such as early GI symptoms and miosis.

It should be re-emphasized that mustard reacts with tissue within minutes of entering the body and that blood, tissue, and blister fluid do not contain free mustard, nor do they represent a contamination risk for medical personnel.

CLINICAL EFFECTS

Topical effects of mustard occur in the eye, airways, and skin. Systemically absorbed mustard may produce effects in the bone marrow, GI tract, and CNS. Direct injury to the GI tract may also occur following ingestion of the compound.

Combined data from U.S. forces in World War I and Iranians in the Iraq-Iran conflict suggest equal incidence of eye, airway, and skin involvement (between 80 and 90% for each). However, there were higher incidences of eye and lung damage in Iranian casualties than in World War I casualties, probably because of the larger amount of evaporation of the agent in the hot climate.

Skin. Erythema is the mildest and earliest form of skin injury after exposure to mustard. It resembles sunburn and is associated with pruritus or burning, stinging pain. Erythema begins to appear in 2 to 48 hours after vapor exposure with time of onset dependent on Ct, ambient temperature and humidity, and skin site exposed. The skin sites most sensitive are the warm, moist locations with thinner skin such as the perineum, external genitalia, axillae, antecubital fossae, and neck.

Within the erythematous areas, small vesicles can develop which may later coalesce to form bullae. The typical bulla, or blister, is large, dome-shaped, thin-walled, translucent, yellowish, and surrounded by erythema. The blister fluid is clear, at first thin and straw-colored, but later yellowish and tending to coagulate. The fluid does not contain mustard and is not a vesicant.

At extremely high doses such as those from liquid exposure, lesions may develop a central zone of coagulation necrosis with blister formation at the periphery. These lesions take longer to heal and are more prone to secondary infection than the uncomplicated lesions seen at lower exposure levels.

Pulmonary. The primary airway lesion from mustard is necrosis of the mucosa with later damage to the musculature of the airways if the amount of agent is large. The damage begins in the upper airways and descends to the lower airways in a dose-dependent manner. Usually the terminal airways and alveoli are affected only as a terminal event. Pulmonary edema is not usually present unless the damage is very severe, and then it usually is hemorrhagic.

The earliest effects from mustard, perhaps the only effects from a low Ct, involve the nose, sinuses, and pharynx. There may be irritation or burning of the nares, epistaxis, sinus pain or irritation, and irritation or soreness of the pharynx. As the Ct increases, other effects occur - laryngitis with voice changes and a nonproductive cough. Damage to the trachea and upper bronchi leads to a cough productive of sputum. Lower airway involvement causes dyspnea and an increasingly severe cough with increased quantities of sputum. Terminally, there may be necrosis of the smaller airways with hemorrhagic edema into surrounding alveoli. This hemorrhagic pulmonary edema is rarely a feature.

Necrosis of the airway mucosa with resulting inflammation can cause pseudomembrane formation. Pseudomembranes may occur from the most proximal parts of the airways to the most distal portions. These membranes may cause local airway obstruction at the sites of formation, and detachment may lead to obstruction of lower airways.

The cause of death in mustard poisoning is commonly respiratory failure. Mechanical obstruction by pseudomembranes and agent-induced laryngospasm are important causes of death in the first 24 hours after exposure. Deaths occurring from the third to the sixth day after exposure result from secondary bacterial pneumonia caused by bacterial invasion of denuded respiratory mucosa and necrotic debris. Agent-induced bone marrow suppression is a contributory factor in later, septic deaths from pneumonia.

Eyes. The eyes are the organs most sensitive to mustard vapor injury. The latent period is shorter for eye injury than for skin injury and is also Ct dependent.

After low-dose vapor exposure, irritation evidenced by reddening of the eyes may be the only effect. As the dose increases, the spectrum of injury includes progressively more severe conjunctivitis, photophobia, blepharospasm, pain, and corneal damage.

Blisters do not normally form in the eyes. Instead, swelling and loosening of corneal epithelial cells lead to corneal edema and clouding with leukocytes (which affects vision). Corneal vascularization with secondary edema may last for weeks. Scarring between the iris and lens may follow severe effects; this scarring may restrict pupillary movements and may predispose victims to glaucoma.

The most severe damage is caused by liquid mustard from airborne droplets or by self-contamination. After extensive eye exposure, severe corneal damage with possible perforation of the cornea and loss of the eye can occur. Eye loss also results from panophthalmitis if appropriate therapy is not instituted.

During World War I, mild conjunctivitis accounted for 75% of eye injuries, with recovery in one to two weeks. Moderate conjunctivitis with minimal corneal involvement, blepharospasm, edema of the lids and conjunctivae, and orange-peel roughening of the cornea accounted for 15% of the cases, with recovery in four to six weeks. Severe corneal involvement accounted for 10% of the cases. Those with permanent corneal damage accounted for less than 1% of cases. About 0.1% of these severe casualties would meet the criteria for legal blindness today.

Miosis noted after mustard exposure in both humans and experimental animals is probably from the cholinomimetic activity of mustard.

<u>Gastrointestinal (GI) tract</u>. The mucosa of the GI tract is very susceptible to mustard damage, either from systemic absorption or ingestion of the agent. However, reports of severe GI effects from mustard poisoning are relatively infrequent.

Mustard exposure, even exposure to a small amount, will often cause nausea, with or without vomiting, lasting 24 hours or less. The nausea and vomiting appear not to be a direct effect of the agent on the GI tract, but rather they are from a stress reaction, a nonspecific reaction to the odor, or cholinergic stimulation by mustard. Further GI symptoms are usually minimal unless the exposure was severe (even then, GI signs are not common) or exposure resulted from ingestion of contaminated food or drink. Diarrhea has been reported; constipation is equally common. Diarrhea (rarely bloody) and vomiting beginning days after a high-dose exposure imply a poor prognosis.

__Central nervous system (CNS).__ The CNS effects of mustard remain poorly defined. Animal work demonstrated that mustards (particularly the nitrogen mustards) are convulsants, and there are several human case reports describing victims who were exposed to very large amounts and had neurological effects within several hours after exposure just prior to death. Reports from World War I, and again from Iran, described people exposed to small amounts of mustard who appeared sluggish, apathetic, and lethargic. These reports suggest that minor psychological problems could linger for a year or longer.

TIME COURSE OF EFFECTS

Mustard binds irreversibly to tissue within several minutes after contact. If decontamination is not done immediately after exposure, there is no way to prevent injury, although later decontamination might prevent a more severe lesion.

The clinical effects of mustard are delayed. Signs and symptoms may appear as early as 2 hours after a high-dose exposure, whereas following a low-dose vapor exposure, the latent or asymptomatic period may extend to 48 hours. There are several reports of individuals exposed to very large amounts who died within hours; this type of occurrence is extremely rare. The typical onset time is between four and eight hours. The concentration (C) of the mustard vapor, time (t) of exposure, ambient weather, and body site exposed are factors in the onset time.

It must be emphasized that **mustard causes tissue damage within several minutes after contact without causing any concomitant clinical effects**, e.g., burning or erythema. Because of the lack of immediate effects, the contaminated person is often unaware of the exposure and does not decontaminate. **To prevent injury, decontamination must be done immediately after contact**. Later decontamination may prevent further damage, absorption, or spread of the agent.

Table. Effects of Mustard Vapor

ORGAN	SEVERITY	EFFECTS	ONSET OF FIRST EFFECT
Eye	Mild	Tearing, itchy, burning, gritty feeling	4-12 hours
	Moderate	Above, plus reddening, swelling of lids, moderate pain	3-6 hours
	Severe	Marked swelling of lids, possible cornea damage, severe pain	1-2 hours
Airways	Mild	Runny nose, sneezing, nosebleed, hoarseness, hacking cough	12-24 hours
	Severe	Above, plus severe productive cough, shortness of breath	2-4 hours
Skin	Mild to Severe	Erythema (redness), blisters	2-24 hours

DIFFERENTIAL DIAGNOSIS

Of the three vesicant agents, mustard is the only one that does not cause immediate pain. The casualty is asymptomatic until the lesion becomes apparent hours later.

Lewisite and phosgene oxime, in contrast, cause immediate pain or irritation to the eye, skin, or respiratory tract. This causes sufficient stimulus to decontaminate immediately or to mask.

Isolated small blisters or a small group of blisters suggest possible exposure to mustard, to plants such as poison ivy or poison oak, drugs, or other substances. The physical characteristics of the lesion are not distinctive; therefore, the history of exposure is invaluable.

Although the blisters of mustard and Lewisite are slightly different (there is less erythema around the Lewisite blister), this information is of little value in individual cases.

LABORATORY FINDINGS

Leukocytosis occurs during the first day, and the magnitude of increase in leukocytes during the subsequent days correlates roughly with the amount of tissue injury, primarily to skin or pulmonary tissue. If systemic absorption is large, leukocytes in the peripheral blood will decrease beginning on day three to day five; this decrease indicates damage to precursor cells in the blood-forming organs. The fall may be precipitate, e.g., a decrease of 5000 to 10,000 cells/day. If the marrow damage is severe, erythrocytes and thrombocytes may later decrease, but the casualty usually recovers or dies before this is apparent. A leukocyte count of 500 or fewer is a sign of an unfavorable prognosis.

Signs of a chemical pneumonitis may appear within the first two to three days after inhalation exposure. Leukocytosis, fever, and sputum production suggest a bacterial process, but within this time period sputum cultures are usually negative for pathogens. Organisms commonly invade the damaged airway tissue at days three to five. A change in the fever pattern, an increase in leukocytosis, and a change in the character of the sputum in this time period suggest a bacterial process. Sputum Gram Stain and culture should be done for identification of the specific organism.

Damaged skin should be cultured routinely, particularly if there is an increase in the exudate or in the inflammatory reaction.

Although GI bleeding is unusual, declining hematocrit values should prompt serial analyses of stool for occult blood.

Thiodiglycol, a urinary metabolite of sulfur mustard, can be measured by the Theater Army Medical Laboratory (TAML), which will be deployed. There is no clinical laboratory test for mustard in blood or tissue, nor is one expected, as mustard is biotransformed and bound to tissues within minutes after absorption. However, ways to measure blood and tissue adducts produced in the body after reaction with sulfur mustard are being studied.

MEDICAL MANAGEMENT

The management of a patient exposed to mustard may be simple, as in the provision of symptomatic care for a sunburn-like erythema, or extremely complex, as providing total management for a severely ill patient with burns, immunosuppression, and multi-system involvement. Suggested therapeutic measures for each organ system are provided below. Guidelines for general patient care are not intended to take the place of sound clinical judgment, especially in the management of complicated cases.

Skin. Erythema should be treated with calamine or other soothing lotion or cream (e.g., 0.25% camphor and menthol, calamine) to reduce burning and itching. Small blisters (under 1-2 cm) should be left intact, but because larger ones will eventually break (the blister fluid does not contain mustard), they should be carefully unroofed. Denuded areas should be irrigated three to four times daily with saline, another sterile solution, or soapy water and then liberally covered with a topical antibiotic such as silver sulfadiazine or mafenide acetate to a thickness of 1-2 mm. If an antibiotic cream is not available, sterile petrolatum will be useful. Modified Dakins solution (sodium hypochlorite) was used in World War I and in Iranian casualties for irrigation and as an antiseptic.

Multiple or large areas of vesication suggest the need for hospitalization and whirlpool bath irrigation.

Systemic analgesics should be used liberally, particularly before manipulation of the patient or irrigation of the burn areas. Systemic antipruritics such as trimeprazine should be tried if needed. Monitoring of fluids and electrolytes is important in any sick patient, but it must be recognized that fluid loss is not of the magnitude seen with thermal burns. Clinicians accustomed to treating patients with thermal burns must resist the temptation to overhydrate a mustard casualty with a similar amount of burned body surface.

Eyes. Conjunctival irritation from a low Ct will respond to any of a number of available ophthalmic solutions after the eyes are thoroughly irrigated. Regular application of homatropine (or other anticholinergic drug) ophthalmic ointment will reduce or prevent future synechiae formation. A topical antibiotic applied several times a day will reduce the incidence and severity of infection. Vaseline or a similar substance should be applied to the edges of the lids regularly to prevent them from sticking together. This prevents adhesions and later scarring during healing and also permits drainage of any underlying infection or pus. Topical analgesics may be useful initially if blepharospasm is too severe to permit an adequate examination, but topical analgesics should otherwise be avoided and systemic analgesics should be given for eye pain. Topical steroids are not of proven value, but their use during the first day or two might reduce inflammation. Further use should be relegated to an ophthalmologist. Sunglasses may reduce discomfort from photophobia.

The patient should be constantly reassured that complete healing and restoration of vision will be the outcome.

Pulmonary. Upper airway symptoms (sore throat, nonproductive cough, and hoarseness) may respond to steam inhalation and cough suppressants. Although a productive cough and dyspnea accompanied by fever and leukocytosis occurring 12 to 24 hours after exposure may suggest a bacterial process to the clinician, he must resist the urge to use antibiotics for this process, which in fact is a sterile bronchitis or pneumonitis. Infection often occurs on about the third day. Its presence is signaled by an increased fever, an increase in the pulmonary infiltrate by x-ray, and an increase in sputum production and a change in sputum character to purulent. Appropriate antibiotic therapy should await confirmation of the clinical impression by positive sputum studies (Gram stain and culture).

Intubation should be performed early before laryngeal spasm or edema make it difficult or impossible. Intubation permits better ventilation and facilitates suction of the necrotic and inflammatory debris. Oxygen may be needed, and early use of PEEP or CPAP may be of benefit. If there is a suggestion of pseudomembrane formation, bronchoscopy should be done to permit suctioning of the necrotic debris by direct vision.

Bronchodilators may be of benefit for bronchospasm. If they fail, steroids may be tried. There is little evidence that the routine use of steroids is beneficial. The need for continuous use of assisted or controlled ventilation suggests a poor prognosis.

Death often occurs between the fifth and tenth day after exposure because of pulmonary insufficiency and infection complicated by a compromised immune response from agent-induced bone marrow damage.

Gastrointestinal. Atropine (0.4-0.6 mg, IM or IV), another anticholinergic drug or antiemetic, should control the early nausea and vomiting. Prolonged vomiting or voluminous diarrhea beginning days after exposure suggests direct involvement of the GI tract by severe systemic poisoning, a poor prognostic sign.

Bone marrow. Sterilization of the gut by nonabsorbable antibiotics should be considered to reduce the possibility of sepsis from enteric organisms. Cellular replacement (bone marrow transplants or transfusions) may be successful, as intact mustard does not persist beyond the few minutes following absorption and would not damage the new cells.

General. A patient severely ill from mustard poisoning requires the general supportive care provided for any severely ill patient, as well as the specific care given to a burn patient. Liberal use of systemic analgesics and antipruritics, as needed, maintenance of fluid and electrolyte balance, and other supportive measures are necessary. Parenteral food supplements including vitamins may also be helpful.

Other. Sulfur donors such as sodium thiosulfate decreased systemic effects and elevated the LD_{50} when given before exposure or within 20 minutes after exposure in experimental animals. Activated charcoal given orally to casualties was of no value. Hemodialysis was not only ineffective, but was actually harmful in several casualties. The rapid biotransformation of the mustard molecule suggests that none of these measures would be beneficial hours or days after exposure.

TRIAGE

Most mustard casualties will be triaged as **delayed**. Those with skin lesions covering several percent to 50% of the BSA will require further medical care but do not need immediate lifesaving assistance. (In contrast, patients with thermal burns covering 20 to 70% of their BSA are considered immediate because of their fluid requirements.) Those with mild to moderate pulmonary effects will also eventually require further care, but are not in the immediate category for triage. Eye injuries from other causes require immediate care, but by the time the mustard eye lesion develops, there is no possibility of reducing the injury. These casualties are also in the delayed category.

Patients with skin lesions covering a small percent of BSA (under 5%), when the lesions are not in vital areas (a burn on the face might prevent mask donning), are triaged as **minimal**. Clinical judgement should dictate whether these patients should be evacuated for care or whether they can return to duty. The tactical situation will also be a factor in the decision. Patients with minor eye injuries to include irritation and reddening can be treated and returned to duty. Those with slight upper respiratory complaints of a hacking cough and an irritated throat which developed 12 hours or longer after exposure might be given symptomatic therapy and returned to duty.

The only mustard casualties who might be triaged as **immediate** are those with moderately severe to severe pulmonary signs and symptoms. Two factors should temper this decision. (1) Casualties who develop severe pulmonary effects within four to six hours of exposure will probably not survive despite maximal medical care, and it might be better to expend limited medical resources elsewhere. (2) If evacuation to a maximal medical care facility is required, the casualty may survive the lengthy trip, but during the delay his lesion may progress to an irreversible stage.

A mustard casualty who has severe pulmonary effects that developed within four to six hours of exposure should be triaged as **expectant**. A casualty who has over 50% BSA burns from mustard liquid might also be categorized as expectant, but this decision would depend on available medical resources at the far rear echelons of medical care. (The LD_{50} for liquid mustard is about 7 grams, or between one and one and a half teaspoons of liquid. This amount will cover about 25% BSA, so an individual with a 50% BSA burn could possibly have two LD_{50}s on his skin. This person might be saved, but at great expenditure of medical resources.)

RETURN TO DUTY

Casualties with minor skin, eye, or pulmonary injuries might be returned to duty as soon as they are given symptomatic therapy at a medical facility. The range of return to duty times for those with more severe but treatable injuries is from one week to a year or longer.

Those with eye injuries should recover in one to three weeks, except for the low percentage of casualties with severe injuries or complications. Casualties with mild to moderate pulmonary injuries should return in a week to a month. Healing of mild skin lesions will enable the casualty to return within several weeks, but patients with large skin lesions will require hospitalization for many months.

LONG-TERM EFFECTS

Repeated symptomatic exposures to mustard over a period of years (as in manufacturing workers) seem to be well established as a causal factor in an increased incidence of upper airway cancer. However, the association between a single exposure to mustard and airway cancer is not well established. A single, severe exposure to mustard may have contributed to other airway problems, such as chronic bronchitis, based on World War I data. A new complication seen in Iranian casualties from the Iran-Iraq War in the 1980s was late-onset tracheobronchial stenosis, which presumably would have been seen in World War I casualties had antibiotic therapy been available to allow those who died from secondary bacterial pneumonia to survive.

Several eye diseases, such as chronic conjunctivitis and delayed keratitis, may follow a single, severe exposure of the eye to mustard. Skin scarring and pigment changes may follow a severe skin lesion from mustard; cancer sometimes develops in scarred skin.

Mustard is classed as a mutagen and carcinogen based on laboratory studies. However, there are no data to implicate mustard as a reproductive toxin in man, and there is no evidence that mustard is a causative factor in nonairway, non-skin cancer in man.

LEWISITE

L

SUMMARY

Signs and Symptoms: Lewisite causes immediate pain or irritation of skin and mucous membranes. Erythema and blisters on the skin and eye and airway damage similar to those seen after mustard exposures develop later.

Detection: M256A1, M272 water testing kit, MINICAMS, the ICAD, M18A2, M21 remote sensing alarm, M90, M93A1 Fox, Bubbler, CAM, and DAAMS (but **NOT** the M8A1 automatic chemical agent alarm), M8 paper, or M9 paper.

Decontamination: M291, 0.5% hypochlorite, water in large amounts.

Management: immediate decontamination; symptomatic management of lesions the same as for mustard lesions; a specific antidote (BAL) will decrease systemic effects.

OVERVIEW

Lewisite is a vesicant that damages the eyes, skin, and airways by direct contact. After absorption, it causes an increase in capillary permeability to produce hypovolemia, shock, and organ damage. Exposure to Lewisite causes immediate pain or irritation, although lesions require hours to become full-blown. Management of a Lewisite casualty is similar to management of a mustard casualty, although a specific antidote, British-Anti-Lewisite (BAL, dimercaprol), will alleviate some effects.

HISTORY/MILITARY RELEVANCE

Dr. Wilford Lee Lewis first synthesized Lewisite in 1918, but production was too late for its use in World War I. It has not been used in warfare, although some countries may stockpile it. Lewisite is sometimes mixed with mustard to achieve a lower freezing point of the mixture for ground dispersal and aerial spraying.

PHYSICOCHEMICAL CHARACTERISTICS

Lewisite is an oily, colorless liquid with the odor of geraniums. It is more volatile than mustard.

DETECTION AND PROTECTION

The immediately-dangerous-to-life-and-health (IDLH) concentration of Lewisite (L) is 0.003 mg/m^3. The M8A1 automatic chemical-agent detector alarm is incapable of detecting Lewisite. However, liquid Lewisite turns M8 paper a ketchup red, and M9 paper will turn pink, red, reddish-brown, or purple when exposed to liquid nerve agents or vesicants, but does not specifically identify either the class of agent or the specific agent. The detectors in the chart below can detect Lewisite (L) at the threshold limits given.

DETECTOR	L
M256A1	14.0 mg/min^3
M272 (in water)	2.0 mg/min^3
MINICAMS	0.0006 mg/min^3
ICAD	10.0 mg/min^3
M18A2	10.0 mg/min^3
M21	150.0 mg/min^3
M90	0.2 mg/min^3
M93A1 Fox	10 - 100 mcg/l
Bubbler	0.003 mg/min^3
CAM	2.0 mg/min^3
DAAMS	0.003 mg/min^3

Because the odor of Lewisite may be faint or lost after accommodation, olfactory detection of the odor of geraniums is not a reliable indicator of Lewisite exposure. The activated charcoal in the canister of the chemical protective mask adsorbs Lewisite, as does the charcoal in the chemical protective overgarment. Lewisite attacks the butyl rubber in the chemical protective gloves and boots, which nevertheless are expected to protect against field concentrations of Lewisite until they can be exchanged for fresh gloves and boots. Proper wear of the chemical protective mask and chemical protective ensemble affords full protection against Lewisite.

MECHANISM OF TOXICITY

Lewisite is readily absorbed from the skin, eyes, and respiratory tract, as well as by ingestion and via wounds. It is systemically distributed to almost all organs and tissues of the body where it participates in a variety of chemical reactions. It is eventually eliminated primarily as reaction products in the urine.

TOXICITY

Lewisite causes nasal irritation at a Ct of about 8 $mg\text{-}min/m^3$, and its odor is noted at a Ct of about 20 $mg\text{-}min/m^3$. Lewisite causes vesication and death from inhalation at the same Ct as mustard. Liquid

Lewisite causes vesication at about 14 mcg, and the LD_{50} of liquid Lewisite applied to the skin is about 2.8 grams.

TOXICODYNAMICS (MECHANISM OF ACTION)

Although Lewisite contains trivalent arsenic and combines with thiol groups in many enzymes, its exact mechanism of biological activity is unknown.

CLINICAL EFFECTS

Organ Systems. Unlike mustard, Lewisite vapor or liquid causes immediate pain or irritation. A person with a droplet of Lewisite on his skin will note the burning and will immediately take steps to try and remove it. The vapor is so irritating that a person will seek to mask or leave the contaminated area if possible. Because this warning causes the person exposed to take immediate steps to decontaminate, the Lewisite lesion will probably not be as severe as the lesion from mustard, as exposure to mustard is often undetected and decontamination is not done.

There are almost no data on humans exposed to Lewisite. The following information is based on animal investigations.

Skin. Within about five minutes after contact, liquid Lewisite will produce a grayish area of dead epithelium. Erythema and blister formation follow more rapidly than in a similar lesion from mustard, although the full lesion does not develop for 12 to 18 hours. The lesion has more tissue necrosis and tissue sloughing than does a mustard lesion.

Eyes. Lewisite causes pain and blepharospasm on contact. Edema of the conjunctiva and lids follows, and the eyes may be swollen shut within an hour. Iritis and corneal damage may follow if the dose is high. Liquid Lewisite causes severe eye damage within minutes of contact.

Respiratory. The extreme irritancy of Lewisite to the nasal area and upper airways causes the person to mask or exit the area. Scanty data indicate that Lewisite causes the same airway signs and symptoms as does mustard. The airway mucosa is the primary target, and damage progresses down the airways in a dose-dependent manner. Pseudomembrane formation is prominent. Pulmonary edema, which occurs rarely and usually only to a minimal degree after mustard exposure, may complicate exposure to Lewisite.

Other. Available data suggest that Lewisite causes an increase in permeability of systemic capillaries with resulting intravascular fluid loss, hypovolemia, shock, and organ congestion. This may lead to hepatic or renal necrosis with more prominent GI effects (including vomiting and diarrhea) than after mustard.

<u>Physical Findings</u>. The findings are similar to those caused by mustard. As noted, the tissue damage at the site of the skin lesion may be more severe.

TIME COURSE OF EFFECTS

Pain and irritation from either liquid or vapor Lewisite are immediate. Early tissue destruction is more obvious than after mustard, but the lesion is not full-blown for 12 hours or longer.

DIFFERENTIAL DIAGNOSIS

Although differences have been reported between the skin lesions from mustard and Lewisite (less surrounding erythema and more tissue destruction characterize Lewisite blisters), these are of little diagnostic assistance in a single patient. The history of immediate pain on contact is absent after mustard exposure and present after Lewisite or phosgene oxime exposures.

Other substances cause erythema and blisters, and often the history of exposure is the most helpful tool in diagnosis.

LABORATORY FINDINGS

There is no specific diagnostic test for Lewisite. Leukocytosis, fever, and other signs of tissue destruction will occur.

MEDICAL MANAGEMENT

Early decontamination is the only way of preventing or lessening Lewisite damage. Since this must be accomplished within minutes after exposure, this is self-aid rather than medical management.

The guidelines for the management of a mustard casualty will be useful. Lewisite does not cause damage to hematopoietic organs as mustard does; however, fluid loss from the capillaries necessitates careful attention to fluid balance.

British Anti-Lewisite (BAL, dimercaprol) was developed as an antidote for Lewisite and is used in medicine as a chelating agent for heavy metals. There is evidence that BAL in oil, given intramuscularly, will reduce the systemic effects of Lewisite. However, BAL itself causes some toxicity, and the user should read the package insert carefully. British-Anti-Lewisite skin and ophthalmic ointment decreases the severity of skin and eye lesions when applied immediately after early decontamination; however, neither is currently manufactured.

TRIAGE

Casualties should be triaged using the guidelines for triage of mustard patients.

RETURN TO DUTY

Casualties with minor skin lesions who receive symptomatic therapy can be returned to duty quickly. Because Lewisite generally causes more tissue damage than mustard, casualties with eye and larger skin lesions should be triaged as **delayed** and **evacuated**. Whether to triage those with pulmonary injury as immediate, delayed, or expectant depends on the severity of the injury and how quickly after exposure it occurred.

PHOSGENE OXIME

CX

SUMMARY

Signs and Symptoms: immediate burning and irritation followed by wheal-like skin lesions and eye and airway damage.

Detection: M256A1, M18A2, M90, and M93 Fox (but **NOT** the M272 water testing kit), MINICAMS, the ICAD, M21 remote sensing alarm, Bubbler, CAM, DAAMS, the M8A1 automatic chemical agent alarm, M8 paper, or M9 paper.

Decontamination: water in large amounts, 0.5% hypochlorite, M291.

Management: immediate decontamination, symptomatic management of lesions.

OVERVIEW

Phosgene oxime (CX) is an urticant or nettle agent that causes a corrosive type of skin and tissue lesion. It is not a true vesicant since it does not cause blisters. The vapor is extremely irritating, and both the vapor and liquid cause almost immediate tissue damage upon contact. There is very scanty information available on CX.

MILITARY SIGNIFICANCE

There is no current assessment of the potential of CX as a military threat agent.

PHYSICOCHEMICAL CHARACTERISTICS

Phosgene oxime is a solid at temperatures below 95°F, but the vapor pressure of the solid is high enough to produce symptoms. Traces of many metals cause it to decompose; however, it corrodes most metals.

DETECTION AND PROTECTION

The immediately-dangerous-to-life-and-health (IDLH) concentration of CX has not been defined. The M272 water testing kit, MINICAMS, ICAD, M21 remote sensing alarm, CAM, ACAMS, DAAMS, and M8A1 automatic chemical-agent detector alarm are incapable of detecting CX. Likewise, M8 and M9 paper should not be depended upon to detect this agent. The M256A1 detector ticket reacts to the presence of CX, but the detection threshold is not known with certainty. The detectors in the following chart are capable of detecting CX at the threshold limits given.

DETECTOR	CX
M18A2	0.5 mg/min^3
M90	0.15 mg/min^3
M93A1 Fox	10 - 100 mcg/l

Because the odor of phosgene may be faint or lost after accommodation, olfactory detection of a pepperish or pungent odor is not a reliable indicator of the presence of CX. The activated charcoal in the canister of the chemical protective mask adsorbs CX, as does the charcoal in the chemical protective overgarment. Phosgene oxime may attack the butyl rubber in the chemical protective gloves and boots, which nevertheless are expected to protect against field concentrations of CX until they can be exchanged for fresh gloves and boots. Proper wear of the chemical protective mask and chemical protective ensemble affords full protection against CX.

MECHANISM OF TOXICITY

The toxicokinetics of CX are not known in detail. Penetration of exposed surfaces is rapid, and systemic distribution to most organs and tissues, including the GI tract, is probably important.

TOXICITY

The estimated LCt_{50} by inhalation is 1500-2000 mg·min/m^3. The LD_{50} for skin exposure has been estimated as 25 mg/kg.

TOXICODYNAMICS (MECHANISM OF ACTION)

The mechanism by which CX causes biological effects is unknown.

CLINICAL EFFECTS

Skin. Phosgene oxime liquid or vapor causes pain on contact, which is followed in turn by blanching with an erythematous ring in 30 seconds, a wheal in

30 minutes, and necrosis later. The extreme pain may persist for days.

Eyes. Phosgene oxime is extremely painful to the eyes. The damage is probably similar to that caused by Lewisite.

Pulmonary. Phosgene oxime is very irritating to the upper airways. This agent causes pulmonary edema after inhalation and after skin application.

Other. Some animal data suggest that CX may cause hemorrhagic inflammatory changes in the GI tract.

TIME COURSE OF EFFECTS

Phosgene oxime causes immediate pain and irritation to all exposed skin and mucous membranes. The time course of damage to other tissue probably parallels that of damage to the skin.

DIFFERENTIAL DIAGNOSIS

Other causes of urticaria and skin necrosis must be considered. Common urticants do not cause the extreme pain that CX does.

LABORATORY FINDINGS

There are no distinctive laboratory findings.

MEDICAL MANAGEMENT

Management is supportive. The skin lesion should be managed in the same way that a necrotic ulcerated lesion from another cause would be managed.

TRIAGE

Because of the continuing pain, most casualties should be placed in the **delayed** category and evacuated.

RETURN TO DUTY

The decision to return a CX casualty to duty should be based on healing of the lesion(s) and the casualty's freedom from discomfort.

NERVE AGENTS
GA, GB, GD, GF, VX

SUMMARY

Signs and Symptoms:

Vapor:

Small exposure -- miosis, rhinorrhea, mild difficulty breathing.

Large exposure -- sudden loss of consciousness, convulsions, apnea, flaccid paralysis, copious secretions, miosis.

Liquid on skin:

Small to moderate exposure -- localized sweating, nausea, vomiting, feeling of weakness.

Large exposure -- sudden loss of consciousness, convulsions, apnea, flaccid paralysis, copious secretions.

Detection: M256A1, CAM, M8 paper, M9 paper, M8A1 and M8 alarm systems.

Decontamination: M291, M258A1, hypochlorite, large amounts of water.

Immediate management: administration of MARK I Kits (atropine and pralidoxime chloride); diazepam in addition if casualty is severe; ventilation and suction of airways for respiratory distress.

OVERVIEW

Nerve agents are the most toxic of the known chemical agents. They are hazards in their liquid and vapor states and can cause death within minutes after exposure. Nerve agents inhibit acetylcholinesterase in tissue, and their effects are caused by the resulting excess acetylcholine.

HISTORY/MILITARY RELEVANCE

Nerve agents were developed in pre-World War II Germany. Germany had stockpiles of nerve agent munitions during World War II, but did not use them for reasons that are still unclear. In the closing days of the war, the U.S. and its allies discovered these stockpiles, developed the agents, and manufactured nerve agent munitions. The U.S.' chemical agent stockpile contains the nerve agents sarin (GB) and VX.

Nerve agents are considered major military threat agents. The only known battlefield use of nerve agents was in the Iraq-Iran conflict. Intelligence analysts indicate that many countries have the technology to manufacture nerve agent munitions.

PHYSICAL CHARACTERISTICS

Nerve agents are liquids under temperate conditions. When dispersed, the more volatile ones constitute both a vapor and a liquid hazard. Others are less volatile and represent primarily a liquid hazard. The "G-agents" are more volatile than VX. Sarin (GB) is the most volatile, but it evaporates less readily than water. GF is the least volatile of the G-agents.

Nerve agents can be dispersed from missiles, rockets, bombs, howitzer shells, spray tanks, land mines, and other large munitions.

DETECTION AND PROTECTION

The IDLH (immediately-dangerous-to-life-and-health concentrations of nerve agents are 0.0001 mg/m^3 for tabun (GA), 0.0001 mg/m^3 for sarin (GB), 0.0003 mg/m^3 for soman (GD), 0.0001 mg/m^3 for GF, and 0.0001 mg/m^3 for VX. Liquid G agents turn M8 paper a "gold" yellow, and VX turns M8 paper a "verdana" or "olive" green. M9 paper will turn pink, red, reddish brown, or purple when exposed to liquid nerve agents or vesicants but does not specifically identify either the class of agent or the specific agent.

The following detectors have the capacity to detect nerve agents at the threshold limits given:

Detector	GA (Tabun)	GB (Sarin)	GD (Soman)	GF	VX
M256A1	Unk.	0.05 mg/m^3	Unk.	Unk.	0.02 mg/m^3
M272 (in water)	0.02 mg/m^3	0.02 mg/m^3	0.02 mg/m^3		0.02 mg/m^3
MINI-CAMS		0.0001 mg/m^3	0.001 ppbv		0.00001 mg/m^3
ICAD	0.5 mg/m^3	0.5 mg/m^3	0.5 mg/m^3		
M18A2		0.02 mg/m^3			0.1 mg/m^3
M21	3.0 mg/m^3	3.0 mg/m^3	3.0 mg/m^3		
M90	0.04 mg/m^3	0.04 mg/m^3	0.04 mg/m^3	0.04 mg/m^3	0.04 mg/m^3
M93A1 Fox		62 mg/m^3	0.1-1 mcg/l		1-10 mcg/l
ACAMS		0.0001 mg/m^3			0.00001 mg/m^3
Bubbler		0.0001 mg/m^3			0.00001 mg/m^3
CAM	0.03 mg/m^3	0.03 mg/m^3	0.03 mg/m^3	0.03 mg/m^3	0.01 mg/m^3
DAAMS		0.0001 mg/m^3			0.0001 mg/m^3

Because the odor of nerve agents may be faint or lost after accommodation, olfactory detection of the odor of fruit or fish is not a reliable indicator of mustard exposure. The activated charcoal in the canister of the chemical protective mask absorbs nerve agents present as vapor or gas, as does the charcoal in the chemical protective overgarment; and the butyl rubber in the chemical protective gloves and boots is impermeable to nerve agents. Proper wear of the protective mask and the chemical protective ensemble affords full protection against nerve agents.

MECHANISM OF TOXICITY

Nerve agents are organophosphorous cholinesterase inhibitors. They inhibit the butyrylcholinesterase in the plasma, acetylcholinesterase on the red cell, and acetylcholinesterase at cholinergic receptor sites in tissue. The three enzymes are not the same; even the two acetylcholinesterases have slightly different properties, although both have a high affinity for acetylcholine. The blood enzymes provide an estimate of the tissue enzyme activity. After acute exposure to a nerve agent, the erythrocyte enzyme activity most closely reflects the activity of the tissue enzyme, but during recovery the plasma enzyme activity more closely parallels tissue enzyme activity.

After a nerve agent inhibits the tissue enzyme, the enzyme cannot hydrolyze acetylcholine, the neurotransmitter, at cholinergic receptor sites. Acetylcholine accumulates and continues to stimulate the affected organ. The clinical effects from nerve agent exposure are caused by excess acetylcholine.

The attachment of the agent to the enzyme is permanent (unless removed by therapy). Erythrocyte enzyme activity returns at the rate of erythrocyte turnover, about 1% per day. Tissue and plasma enzyme activities return with synthesis of new enzymes. The rate of return of the tissue and plasma enzymes is not the same, nor is the rate the same for all tissue enzymes. However, the agent can be removed from the enzyme and the enzyme "reactivated" by several types of compounds, the most useful of which are the oximes. If the agent-enzyme complex has not "aged," oximes are useful therapeutically. Aging is a biochemical process by which the agent-enzyme complex becomes refractory to oxime reactivation of the enzyme. For most nerve agents, the aging time is longer than the time within which acute casualties will be seen. However, the aging time of the GD-enzyme complex is about two minutes, and the usefulness of oximes in GD poisoning is greatly decreased after this period.

Organs with cholinergic receptor sites include the smooth muscles, skeletal muscles, central nervous system (CNS), and most exocrine glands. In addition, cranial efferents and ganglionic afferents are cholinergic nerves.

Muscarine will stimulate some of the cholinergic sites, and these are known as muscarinic sites. Organs with these sites include the smooth muscles and glands. Nicotine will stimulate other cholinergic sites, known as nicotinic sites, which are those in skeletal muscle and ganglia. The CNS contains both types of receptors, but the pharmacology in the CNS is more complex and less well understood. Atropine and similar compounds block the effects of excess acetylcholine more effectively at muscarinic sites than at nicotinic sites.

Some commonly used pesticides (for example, the organophosphate (OP) Malathion and the carbamate Sevin) and some common therapeutic drugs (the carbamates pyridostigmine [Mestinon] and physostigmine [Antilirium]) also inhibit acetylcholinesterase and can be considered "nerve agents." However, while the OP pesticides cause the same biological effects as nerve agents, there are some important differences in the duration of biological activity and response to therapy.

CLINICAL EFFECTS

The initial effects of exposure to a nerve agent depend on the dose and route of exposure. The initial effects from a sublethal amount of agent by vapor exposure are different than the initial effects from a similar amount of liquid agent on the skin.

Toxicities. The estimated amounts to cause certain effects in man are shown in Tables I and II. In Table I, L indicates lethal, I indicates incapacitating (severe), and M indicates miosis. The large amounts of tabun (GA) and GB required to produce effects after skin application reflect the volatility of these agents. They evaporate rather than penetrate the skin. However, if these agents are occluded and prevented from evaporating, they penetrate the skin very well.

Table I. Vapor Toxicity

mg-min/m³

Agent	LCt_{50}	ICt_{50}	MCt_{50}
GA	400	300	2-3
GB	100	75	3
GD	70	UNK	<1
GF	UNK	UNK	<1
VX	50	35	0.04

Table II. LD_{50} on Skin

Agent	Amount
GA	1000 mg
GB	1700 mg
GD	50 mg
GF	30 mg
VX	10 mg

Sarin (GB), the agent studied most thoroughly in man, will cause miosis, rhinorrhea, and a feeling of tightness in the throat or chest at a Ct of 3 to 5 $mg{\cdot}min/m^3$.

Effects. Exposure to a small amount of nerve agent vapor causes effects in the eyes, nose, and airways. These effects are from local contact of the vapor with the organ and do not indicate systemic absorption of the agent. In this circumstance, the erythrocyte-ChE may be normal or depressed. A small amount of liquid agent on the skin causes systemic effects initially in the gastrointestinal (GI) tract. Lethal amounts of vapor or liquid cause a rapid cascade of events culminating within a minute or two with loss of consciousness and convulsive activity, followed by apnea and muscular flaccidity within several more minutes.

Eye. Miosis is a characteristic sign of exposure to nerve agent vapor. It occurs as a result of direct contact of vapor with the eye. Liquid agent on the skin will not cause miosis if the amount of liquid is small. A moderate amount of liquid may or may not cause miosis. A lethal or near-lethal amount of agent usually causes miosis. A droplet of liquid in or near the eye will also cause miosis. Miosis will begin within seconds or minutes after the onset of exposure to agent vapor, but it may not be complete for many minutes if the vapor concentration is low. Miosis is bilateral in an unprotected individual, but occasionally may be unilateral in a masked person with a leak in his mask eyepiece.

Miosis is often accompanied by complaints of pain, dim vision, blurred vision, conjunctival injection, nausea, and occasionally, vomiting. The pain may be sharp or dull, in or around the eyeball, but more often is a dull ache in the frontal part of the head. Dim vision is due in part to the small pupil, and cholinergic mechanisms in the visual pathways also contribute. The complaint of blurred vision is less easily explained, as objective testing usually indicates an improvement in visual acuity because of the "pin-hole" effect. Conjunctival injection may be mild or severe, and occasionally subconjunctival hemorrhage is present. Nausea (and sometimes vomiting) is part of a generalized complaint of not feeling well. Topical homatropine or atropine in the eye can relieve miosis, pain, dim vision, and nausea.

Nose. Rhinorrhea may be the first indication of nerve agent vapor exposure. Its severity is dose dependent.

Airways. Nerve agent vapor causes bronchoconstriction and increased secretions of the glands in the airways in a dose-related manner. The exposed person may feel a slight tightness in his chest after a small amount of agent and may be in severe distress after a large amount of agent.

Cessation of respiration occurs within minutes after the onset of effects from exposure to a large amount of nerve agent. This apnea is probably mediated through the CNS, although peripheral factors (skeletal muscle weakness, e.g., the intercostal muscles, and bronchoconstriction) may contribute.

Gastrointestinal (GI) tract. After they are absorbed, nerve agents cause an increase in the motility of the GI tract and an increase in secretions by the glands in the wall of the GI tract. Nausea and vomiting are early signs of liquid exposure on the skin. Diarrhea may occur with large amounts of agent.

Glands. Nerve agent vapor causes increases in secretions from the glands it contacts, such as the lacrimal, nasal, salivary, and bronchial glands. Localized sweating around the site of liquid agent on the skin is common, and generalized sweating after a large liquid or vapor exposure is common. Increased secretions of the glands of the GI tract occur after systemic absorption of the agent by either route.

Skeletal muscle. The first effect of nerve agents on skeletal muscle is stimulation producing muscular fasciculations and twitching. After a large amount of agent, fatigue and weakness of muscles are rapidly followed by muscular flaccidity.

Fasciculations are sometimes seen early at the site of a droplet of liquid agent on the skin, and generalized fasciculations are common after a large exposure. These may remain long after most of the other acute signs decrease.

Central nervous system (CNS). The acute CNS signs of exposure to a large amount of nerve agent are loss of consciousness, seizure activity, and apnea. These begin within a minute after exposure to a large amount of agent vapor and may be preceded by an asymptomatic period of 1 to 30 minutes after contact of liquid with the skin.

After exposure to smaller amounts of nerve agents, CNS effects vary and are nonspecific. They may include forgetfulness, an inability to concentrate fully, insomnia, bad dreams, irritability, impaired judgement, and depression. They do not include frank confusion and misperceptions (i.e., hallucinations). These may occur in the absence of physical signs or other symptoms of exposure. After a severe exposure, these symptoms occur upon recovery from the acute severe effects. In either case, they may persist for as long as four to six weeks.

Cardiovascular. The heart rate may be decreased because of stimulation by the vagus nerve, but it is often increased because of other factors such as fright, hypoxia, and the influence of adrenergic stimulation secondary to ganglionic stimulation. Thus, the heart rate may be high, low, or in the normal range. Bradyarrhythmias such as first-, second-, or third-degree heart block may occur. The blood pressure may be elevated from adrenergic factors, but is generally normal until the terminal decline.

PHYSICAL FINDINGS

Physical findings depend on the amount and route of exposure. After exposure to small to moderate amounts of vapor, there are usually miosis and conjunctival injection, rhinorrhea, and pulmonary signs, although the latter may be absent even in the face of mild to moderate pulmonary complaints. In addition to these signs, an exposure to a high Ct may precipitate copious secretions from the nose and mouth, generalized muscular fasciculations, twitching or seizure activity, loss of consciousness, and apnea. Cyanosis, hypotension, and bradycardia may be present just before death.

Exposure to a small droplet of liquid on the skin may produce few physical findings. Sweating, blanching, and occasionally, fasciculations, at the site may be present soon after exposure, but may no longer be present at the onset of GI effects. After a large exposure, the signs are the same as after vapor exposure.

Miosis is a useful sign of exposure to vapor but does not occur after a liquid exposure unless the amount of exposure is large or the exposure is in or close to the eye.

TIME COURSE OF EFFECTS

Effects from nerve agent vapor begin within seconds to several minutes after exposure. Loss of consciousness and onset of seizure activity have occurred within a minute of exposure to a high Ct. After exposure to a very low Ct, miosis and other effects may not begin for several minutes, and miosis may not be complete for 15 to 30 minutes after removal from the vapor. There is no latent period or delay in onset from vapor exposure. Effects may continue to progress for a period of time, but maximal effects usually occur within minutes after exposure stops.

A large amount of liquid on the skin causes effects within minutes. Commonly there is an asymptomatic period of 1 to 30 minutes, and then the sudden onset of an overwhelming cascade of events, including loss of consciousness, seizure activity, apnea, and muscular flaccidity. After small amounts of liquid agent on the skin, the onset of effects has been delayed for as long as 18 hours after contact. These effects are initially gastrointestinal and are usually not life threatening. Generally, the longer the interval, the less severe are the effects.

DIFFERENTIAL DIAGNOSIS

The effects caused by a mild vapor exposure, namely rhinorrhea and tightness in the chest, may easily be confused with an upper respiratory malady or an allergy. Miosis, if present, will help to distinguish these, but the eyes must be examined in very dim light to detect this. Similarly, GI symptoms from another illness may be confused with those from nerve agent effects, and in this instance there will be no useful physical signs. History of possible exposure will be helpful, and laboratory evidence (decreased RBC-ChE activity), if available, will be useful to distinguish the two.

The diagnosis is easier in the severely intoxicated patient. The combination of miosis, copious secretions, and generalized muscular fasciculations in a gasping, cyanotic, and convulsing patient is characteristic.

LABORATORY FINDINGS

Nerve agents inhibit the cholinesterase activity of the blood components, and estimation of this activity is useful in detecting exposure to these agents. The erythrocyte enzyme activity is more sensitive to acute nerve agent exposure than is the plasma enzyme activity.

The amount of inhibition of this enzyme activity does not correlate well with the severity of local effects from mild to moderate vapor exposure. The enzyme activity may be from 0 to 100% of the individual's normal activity in the face of miosis, rhinorrhea, and/or airway symptoms. Normal or nearly normal erythrocyte acetylcholinesterase activity may be present with moderate effects in these organs. At the other extreme, the enzyme may be inhibited by 60 to 70% when miosis or rhinorrhea is the only sign of exposure. Severe systemic effects generally indicate inhibition of the erythrocyte acetylcholinesterase by 70 to 80% or greater.

Other laboratory findings will relate to complications. For example, acidosis may occur after prolonged hypoxia.

MEDICAL MANAGEMENT

Management of a casualty with nerve agent intoxication consists of decontamination, ventilation, administration of the antidotes, and supportive therapy. The condition of the patient dictates the need for each of these and the order in which they are done.

Decontamination is described elsewhere in this manual. Skin decontamination is not necessary after exposure to vapor alone, but clothing should be removed because it may contain "trapped" vapor.

The need for **ventilation** will be obvious, and the means of ventilation will depend on available equipment. Airway resistance is high (50-70 cm of water) because of bronchoconstriction and secretions, and initial ventilation is difficult. The resistance decreases after atropine administration, after which ventilation will be easier. The copious secretions that may be thickened by atropine also impede ventilatory efforts and require frequent suctioning. In reported cases of severe nerve agent exposure, ventilation has been required from 0.5 to 3 hours.

Three drugs are used to treat nerve agent exposure, and another is used as pretreatment for potential nerve agent exposure. The three therapeutic drugs are atropine, pralidoxime chloride, and diazepam. The use of the pretreatment drug pyridostigmine bromide is discussed later in this chapter.

Atropine is a cholinergic blocking or anticholinergic compound. It is extremely effective in blocking the effects of excess acetylcholine at peripheral muscarinic sites. Under experimental conditions, very large amounts may block some cholinergic effects at nicotinic sites, but these antinicotinic effects are not evident even at high clinical doses. When small amounts (2 mg) are given to normal individuals without nerve agent intoxication, atropine causes mydriasis, a decrease in secretions (including a decrease in sweating), mild sedation, a decrease in GI motility, and tachycardia. The amount in three MARK I Kits may cause adverse effects on military performance in a normal person. In people not exposed to nerve agents, amounts of 10 mg or higher may cause delirium. Potentially, the most hazardous effect of inadvertent use of atropine (2 mg, IM) in a young person not exposed to a cholinesterase inhibiting compound in a warm or hot atmosphere is inhibition of sweating, which may lead to heat injury. In the military, atropine is packaged in autoinjectors, each containing 2 mg.

Pralidoxime chloride (Protopam chloride, 2-PAMCl) is an oxime. Oximes attach to the nerve agent that is inhibiting the cholinesterase and break the agent-enzyme bond to restore the normal activity of the enzyme. Clinically, this is noticeable in those organs with nicotinic receptors. Abnormal activity in skeletal muscle decreases and normal strength returns. The effects of an oxime are not apparent in organs with muscarinic receptors; oximes do not cause a decrease in secretions, for example. They also are less useful after aging occurs, but with the exception of GD (soman) intoxicated individuals, casualties will be treated before significant aging occurs. Pralidoxime chloride (600 mg) is in an autoinjector for self-use along with the atropine injector. These atropine and pralidoxime chloride autoinjectors are packaged together in a MARK I Kit. Each soldier is issued three MARK I Kits.

Diazepam is an anticonvulsant drug used to decrease convulsive activity and reduce the brain damage caused by prolonged seizure activity. Without the use of pyridostigmine pretreatment, experimental animals died quickly after superlethal doses of nerve agents despite conventional therapy. With pyridostigmine pretreatment (followed by conventional therapy), animals survived superlethal doses of soman but had prolonged periods of seizure activity before recovery. They later had performance decrements and anatomic lesions in their brains. The administration of diazepam with other standard therapy to soman-poisoned animals pretreated with pyridostigmine reduced the seizure activity and its sequelae. Current military doctrine is to administer diazepam with other therapy (three MARK I Kits) at the onset of severe effects from a nerve agent, whether or not seizure activity is among those effects. Each soldier carries one autoinjector containing 10 mg of diazepam for his buddy to administer to him (if he could self-administer it, he would not need it). **Diazepam should be administered**

with the three MARK I Kits when the casualty's condition warrants the use of three kits at the same time. Medical personnel can administer more diazepam to a casualty if necessary. The medical corpsman carries extra diazepam injectors and is authorized to administer two additional injectors at ten-minute intervals to a convulsing casualty.

The doctrine for **self-aid** for nerve agent intoxication states that if an individual has effects from the agent, he/she should self-administer one MARK I Kit. If there is no improvement in ten minutes, he/she should seek out a buddy to assist in the evaluation of his/her condition before further MARK I Kits are given. If a buddy finds an individual severely intoxicated (e.g., gasping respirations, twitching, etc.) so that the individual cannot self-administer a MARK I Kit, the buddy should administer three MARK I Kits and diazepam immediately. The discussion below is advice for medical assistance.

The appropriate number of MARK I Kits to administer initially to a casualty from nerve agent vapor depends on the severity of the effects. Systemic atropine will not reverse miosis (unless administered in very large amounts), and miosis alone is not an indication for a MARK I Kit. If the eye or head pain and nausea associated with the miosis are severe, topical application of atropine (or homatropine) in the eye will bring relief. Topical atropine should not be used without good reason (severe pain), because it causes blurred vision for a day or longer. A casualty with miosis and rhinorrhea should be given one MARK I Kit only if the rhinorrhea is severe and troublesome (he cannot keep his mask on because of fluid). A casualty with mild to moderate dyspnea should be given one or two MARK I Kits, depending on the severity of his distress and the time between exposure and therapy. Some of the respiratory distress from a mild exposure will spontaneously decrease within 15 to 30 minutes after termination of exposure, so if the casualty is not severely uncomfortable, only one MARK I Kit should be used initially. Atropine is quite effective, and care should be taken not to give too much in a casualty who does not need it.

A severe casualty from nerve agent vapor has miosis, copious secretions from the nose and mouth, severe difficulty breathing or apnea, possibly some degree of cyanosis, muscular fasciculations, and twitching or convulsive activity, and is unconscious. He should be given three MARK I Kits and diazepam immediately. Ventilation will be needed and should be done via an endotracheal airway if possible. Suctioning of the excessive airway secretions will be necessary to enhance air exchange and will make ventilatory efforts easier. Atropine, 2 mg, should be repeated at three to five-minute intervals and should be titrated to a reduction of secretions and to reduction of ventilatory resistance. When the IV preparation is available, the preferred route of atropine administration is via the IV route, but this route should be avoided until hypoxia is corrected, because intravenously administered atropine in hypoxic animals has produced ventricular fibrillation. In a hypotensive patient or a patient with poor veins, atropine might be given intratracheally, either via the endotracheal tube or directly into the trachea, for more rapid absorption via the peribronchial vessels.

The medical care provider might err in giving too much atropine to a mild to moderate casualty. More importantly, the care provider might err by giving too little atropine to a severe casualty. In a severe casualty, atropine should be pushed at frequent intervals until secretions are dry (or nearly dry) and until ventilation can be accomplished with ease. In reported cases this has required 10 to 20 mg of atropine within the first several hours. A conscious, less-severely exposed casualty should receive atropine until he is breathing comfortably, and he will be able to communicate this. Dry secretions need not be an endpoint in mild to moderate casualties.

The casualty with skin exposure to liquid is more difficult to evaluate and manage than is a vapor exposure casualty. Agent on the surface of the skin can be decontaminated, but agent absorbed into the skin cannot be removed. The initial effects from absorbed liquid agent can start two to three hours after thorough decontamination of agent droplets on the skin. A casualty from liquid exposure on the skin may continue to worsen because of continued absorption of the agent from the skin depot.

The first effects of a liquid droplet on the skin are sweating with or without blanching, and occasionally, muscular fasciculations at the site. Gastrointestinal effects (nausea, vomiting, and sometimes diarrhea) are the first systemic effects, and these may start from 0.5 to 18 hours after contact with the agent. If these effects occur within the first several hours after exposure, they may portend more severe effects, and initial therapy should be two MARK I Kits. If effects begin later, initial therapy should be one MARK I Kit.

A large amount of liquid agent on the skin will cause effects 1 to 30 minutes after contact, whether or not decontamination was done. Nevertheless, early decontamination may lessen the magnitude of the effects. After a 1 to 30-minute latent or asymptomatic period, the casualty will suddenly lose consciousness and begin seizure activity. The condition of the casualty and management are the same as described for a severe casualty from vapor exposure.

Further care of the severe casualty consists of atropine administration to minimize secretions and ventilation until spontaneous respiration resumes. Oxime administration should be repeated at hourly intervals for two or three additional doses. The preferred method of administration of the oxime is by IV drip of 1 gram over 20 to 30 minutes (more rapid administration will cause hypertension), but 3 additional oxime autoinjectors (total dose of 1.8 grams) may be given if the IV route cannot be used. The need for ventilation may continue for 0.5 to 3 hours. Unless prolonged hypoxia or other complications have occurred, the casualty will eventually begin having spontaneous muscular activity and make sporadic attempts to breathe. Muscles will become stronger and breathing more regular, and the casualty will have intermittent episodes of conscious behavior. Within an hour or two, he will be breathing, moving, and conscious, although he will be weak and intermittently obtunded.

Table III. Nerve Agent Effects
Vapor Exposure

Mild

- Eyes: miosis, dim vision, headache
- Nose: rhinorrhea
- Mouth: salivation
- Lungs: dyspnea ("tightness in the chest")

- Time of onset: seconds to minutes after exposure
- **Self-aid**: one MARK I Kit
- **Buddy-aid**: stand by

<u>**Severe**</u>

- All of the above, plus
- Severe breathing difficulty or cessation of respiration
- Generalized muscular twitching, weakness, or paralysis
- Convulsions
- Loss of consciousness
- Loss of bladder, bowel control
- Time of onset: seconds to minutes after exposure
- **Self-aid**: None - soldier will be unable to help self
- **Buddy-aid**: 3 MARK I Kits and diazepam <u>immediately</u>

Table IV. Nerve Agent Effects
Liquid on Skin

Mild/moderate

- Muscle twitching at site of exposure
- Sweating at site of exposure
- Nausea, vomiting
- Feeling of weakness
- Time of onset: 10 minutes to 18 hours after exposure
- **Self-aid**: one to two MARK I Kits, depending on severity of symptoms
- **Buddy-aid**: stand by

Severe

All of the above, plus

- Severe breathing difficulty or cessation of breathing
- Generalized muscular twitching, weakness, or paralysis

- Convulsions

- Loss of consciousness

- Loss of bladder and bowel control

- Time of onset: minutes to an hour after exposure

- **Self-aid**: none - soldier will be unable to help himself

- **Buddy-aid**: three MARK I Kits and diazepam <u>immediately</u>

PRETREATMENT

In late 1990, the U.S. military fielded pyridostigmine bromide as a pretreatment for nerve agent exposure. Each individual received a blister pack containing twenty-one 30-mg tablets. The dose regimen is one 30-mg tablet every eight hours. When to start and stop dosing is a division or corps' command decision and is made with the advice of the intelligence, chemical, and medical staffs. To use or to stop the pretreatment is not a local decision, nor is it an individual decision.

When given before soman exposure and when that exposure is followed by the standard MARK I therapy, the use of pretreatment will increase the LD_{50}

several fold over the LD_{50} obtained without the use of the pretreatment. When soman is the nerve agent, the use of pyridostigmine increases survival. When the agent is GB or VX, survival after standard MARK I therapy is essentially the same whether or not pyridostigmine pretreatment is used, i.e., pyridostigmine use provides no benefit in GB or VX poisoning. Current data are not adequate to evaluate the effectiveness of pyridostigmine pretreatment for GA or GF exposure.

Pyridostigmine is not an antidote, and it should not be taken after soman exposure. Its use will not decrease the effects of soman. It is ineffective unless standard MARK I therapy is also used in the appropriate manner.

One consequence of the greater survival from the use of pyridostigmine is prolonged seizure activity and subsequent brain damage in the survivors. The early administration of diazepam will decrease these effects.

About 50 years ago, it was noted that carbamates bind to the active site of cholinesterase in a similar manner to the binding of organophosphorus cholinesterase inhibitors to cholinesterase. Additionally, while the carbamate was attached to the active site, an organophosphorus compound could not attach to the enzyme. The carbamate-enzyme binding, or carbamylation, lasts only for hours, rather than for the lifetime of the enzyme as the organophosphorus compound attachment does. While the enzyme is carbamylated, the active site is protected from attack by other compounds such as organophosphorous cholinesterase inhibitors, including nerve agents. After several hours, the carbamate leaves the enzyme (that is, decarbamylation occurs), and the enzyme becomes completely functional again. Thus, the carbamate provides temporary protection for the enzyme against nerve agent attack.

Over the past several decades, many carbamates have been investigated for their effectiveness in animals and their safety in man. Pyridostigmine was chosen and underwent extensive testing in humans. Investigations indicated that it did not interfere with the performance of military tasks and caused no adverse physiological disturbances. The incidence of side effects from the drug during these studies was reported as fewer than 5%.

Tens of thousands of U.S. troops took pyridostigmine during the recent Gulf War Conflict. The incidence of side effects (primarily gastrointestinal and urinary) was over 50%, but only a few percent of the troops sought medical help because of the severity of these effects. The drug was discontinued in less than 1% of cases.

TRIAGE

A severe nerve agent casualty who is unconscious, convulsing or post-ictal, breathing with difficulty or apneic, and possibly flaccid will survive with appropriate, immediate therapy (including ventilation) if he still has an intact circulation. He should be triaged as **immediate** if that therapy can be provided. If a blood pressure cannot be obtained, he should be considered **expectant**.

The casualty with severe symptoms who is spontaneously breathing, has not lost consciousness, and has not seized has an excellent chance of survival with a minimal amount of therapeutic effort. He should be categorized as **immediate** and given three MARK I Kits and diazepam. He may worsen if his exposure was to liquid, and atropine administration should be repeated at frequent intervals. If he loses consciousness, seizes, and becomes apneic, he will be retriaged, and his further care will depend on available resources.

Casualties who are walking and talking will usually be triaged as **minimal**. If a casualty can walk and talk, he is breathing and his circulation is intact. He would not appear to need immediate, life-saving care. This does not preclude self-administration or medic-administration of further antidotes for symptoms, and these should be given as necessary.

A casualty recovering from a severe exposure who has received large amounts of antidotes and has been ventilated will be triaged as **delayed**, because he is in need of further medical observation or care.

RETURN TO DUTY

Return to duty depends on the status of the casualty, his military assignment, and the tactical situation.

Studies indicate that animals with decreased erythrocyte acetylcholinesterase activity from a nerve agent exposure have a decreased LD_{50} for another nerve agent exposure (they are more susceptible to the agent) until that cholinesterase activity returns to at least 75% of its baseline, or pre-exposure activity. Nerve agent exposed workers in a depot or research facility are prevented from returning to work with agents until this recovery occurs. In a battlefield situation, this conservative management should be balanced against the need for the person and his risk of being exposed to a large amount of agent.

In a military field situation, the capability to analyze blood for erythrocyte cholinesterase activity is usually not available, and the "normal" or baseline activity of each individual is not known. The erythrocyte cholinesterase activity in a casualty with severe systemic effects will be inhibited by 70% or greater (30% or less of his pre-exposure activity), and 45 days or longer will be required for cholinesterase activity to return to 75% of pre-exposure activity. The enzyme activity of a casualty with mild or moderate effects from agent vapor might be nearly normal or might be markedly inhibited. A prediction of erythrocyte cholinesterase recovery time is unreliable.

Most individuals triaged as minimal could return to duty within several hours if the tactical situation required all available manpower. The lingering ocular and CNS effects may be limiting factors in these cases. These individuals might be able to fire a rifle, but their performance on a tracking screen might be severely decremented because of both visual problems and difficulty in concentrating. These prolonged effects must be thoroughly evaluated before the casualties are returned to duty. Whether these individuals should be evacuated to a facility with the capability for analysis of erythrocyte cholinesterase activity and retained there until the activity returns will be dictated by the tactical situation.

A casualty who had severe effects might be walking and talking after 6 to 24 hours but will still be unfit for most duties. Ideally, he should be kept under medical observation for a week or longer and not returned until recovery of cholinesterase activity. However, the tactical situation may lead to modification of these guidelines.

LONG-TERM EFFECTS

Minor electroencephalographic changes were noted more than a year after nerve agent exposure when averaged EEGs in a group of people who had been exposed to a nerve agent were compared to a control group. Changes could not be identified in individuals. Neuropsychiatric changes have been noted in individuals for weeks to months after exposure to insecticides.

Polyneuropathy, reported after OP insecticide poisoning, has not been reported in humans exposed to nerve agents and has been produced in animals only at doses of nerve agents so high that survival would be unlikely. The Intermediate Syndrome has not been reported in humans after nerve agent exposure, nor has it been produced in animals by nerve agent administration. Muscular necrosis has been produced in animals after high dose nerve agent exposure but reverses within weeks; it has not been reported in humans.

INCAPACITATING AGENTS
BZ, Agent 15

SUMMARY

Signs and Symptoms: mydriasis; dry mouth; dry skin; increased DTRs; decreased level of concentration; disturbance in perception and interpretation (illusions and/or hallucinations); denial of illness; short attention span; impaired memory.

Detection: No field detector is available.

Decontamination: Gentle, but thorough washing of skin and hair with water or soap and water is required. Bleach is not necessary. Remove clothing.

Management: **Antidote:** physostigmine. **Supportive:** monitoring of vital signs, especially core temperature.

OVERVIEW

BZ is a glycolate anticholinergic compound related to atropine, scopolamine, and hyoscyamine. Dispersal would be as an aerosolized solid (primarily for inhalation) or as agent dissolved in one or more solvents for ingestion or percutaneous absorption. Acting as a competitive inhibitor of acetylcholine at postsynaptic and postjunctional muscarinic receptor sites in smooth muscle, exocrine glands, autonomic ganglia, and the brain, BZ decreases the effective concentration of acetylcholine seen by receptors at these sites. Additionally, BZ causes peripheral nervous system (PNS) effects that in general are the opposite of those seen in nerve agent poisoning. Central nervous system (CNS) effects include stupor, confusion, and confabulation with concrete and panoramic illusions and hallucinations, and with regression to automatic "phantom" behaviors such as plucking and disrobing. The U.S. weaponized BZ, but demilitarization began in 1988 and is complete. Agent 15 is an alleged Iraqi incapacitating agent that is likely to be chemically either identical to BZ or closely related to it. Agent 15 was reportedly stockpiled in large quantities prior to and during the Gulf War. The combination of anticholinergic PNS and CNS effects aids in the diagnosis of patients exposed to these agents. Physostigmine, which increases the concentration of acetylcholine in synapses and in neuromuscular and neuroglandular junctions, is a specific antidote.

HISTORY/MILITARY RELEVANCE

The use of chemicals to induce altered states of mind dates to antiquity and includes the use of plants such as thornapple (*Datura stramonium*) that contain combinations of anticholinergic alkaloids. The use of nonlethal chemicals to render an enemy force incapable of fighting dates back to at least 600 B.C., when Solon's soldiers threw hellebore roots into streams supplying water to enemy troops, who then developed diarrhea. In 184 B.C., Hannibal's army used belladonna plants to induce disorientation, and the Bishop of Muenster in A.D. 1672 attempted to use belladonna-containing grenades in an assault on the city of Groningen. In 1881, members of a railway surveying expedition crossing Tuareg territory in North Africa ate dried dates that tribesmen had apparently deliberately contaminated with *Hyoscyamus falezlez*. In 1908, 200 French soldiers in Hanoi became delirious and experienced hallucinations after being poisoned with a related plant. More recently, accusations of Soviet use of incapacitating agents internally and in Afghanistan were never substantiated.

Following World War II, the U.S. military investigated a wide range of possible nonlethal, psychobehavioral, chemical incapacitating agents to include psychedelic indoles such as lysergic acid diethylamide (LSD-25) and marijuana derivatives, certain tranquilizers, as well as several glycolate anticholinergics. One of the anticholinergic compounds, 3-quinuclidinyl benzilate, was assigned the NATO code BZ and was weaponized beginning in the 1960s for possible battlefield use. Although BZ figured prominently in the plot of the 1990 movie, *Jacob's Ladder,* as the compound responsible for hallucinations and violent deaths in a fictitious American battalion in Vietnam, this agent never saw operational use. Destruction of American stockpiles began in 1988 and is now complete.

In February 1998, the British Ministry of Defence released an intelligence report that accused Iraq of having stockpiled large amounts of a glycolate anticholinergic incapacitating agent known as Agent 15. This compound is speculated either to be identical to BZ or a closely related derivative. Also, in 1998, there were allegations that elements of the Yugoslav People's Army used incapacitating agents against fleeing Bosnian refugees that caused hallucinations and irrational behavior. Physical evidence of BZ use in Bosnia remains elusive, however.

Terms. The term "incapacitation," when used in a general sense, is roughly equivalent to the term "disability" as used in occupational medicine and denotes the inability to perform a task because of a quantifiable physical or mental impairment. In this sense, any of the chemical warfare agents may incapacitate a victim; however, again by the military definition of this type of agent, incapacitation refers to impairments that are temporary and nonlethal. Thus, riot-control agents are incapacitating because they cause temporary loss of vision due to blepharospasm, but they are not considered military incapacitants because the loss of vision does not last long.

Although incapacitation may result from physiological changes such as mucous membrane irritation, diarrhea, or hyperthermia, the term "incapacitating agent" as militarily defined, refers to a compound that produces temporary and nonlethal impairment of military performance by virtue of its psychobehavioral or CNS effects.

Sources other than military. BZ and related anticholinergic compounds can be synthesized in clandestine laboratories, but their illicit use is low possibly because of some unpleasant effects. The anticholinergics atropine, oxybutynin, and scopolamine find use in clinical medicine and are available as pharmaceuticals, as are antihistamines that have prominent anticholinergic side effects. Finally, anticholinergic hallucinogenic compounds are present in plants of the family *Solanaceae*, which include thornapple (Jimson weed, *Datura stramonium*), black henbane (*Hyoscyamus niger*), belladonna (deadly nightshade, *Atropa belladonna*), woody nightshade (*Solanum dulcamara*), and Jerusalem cherry (*Solanum pseudocapsicum*). These plants contain varying proportions of the anticholinergic glycolates atropine, hyoscyamine, and hyoscine. Finally, BZ itself, now called QNB in the scientific community, is widely used in pharmacology as a muscarinic receptor marker.

PHYSICOCHEMICAL CHARACTERISTICS

BZ is the NATO code for 3-quinuclidinyl benzilate (QNB). BZ is odorless. It is stable in most solvents, with a half-life of three to four weeks in moist air; even heat-producing munitions can disperse it. It is extremely persistent in soil and water and on most surfaces. It is also soluble in propylene glycol, DMSO, and other solvents. Agent 15 presumably shares many of the physicochemical properties of BZ.

DETECTION AND PROTECTION

Because BZ is odorless and nonirritating, and because clinical effects are not seen until after a latent period of 30 minutes to 24 hours, exposure could occur without the knowledge of casualties. No currently available field military or civilian detector is designed to disclose the presence of BZ or other anticholinergic compounds in the environment. Confirmation of the exact chemical involved in an incapacitating agent exposure would have to await laboratory analysis of environmental specimens containing the agent. The HEPA filter in the canister of the chemical protective mask prevents exposure of the face and respiratory tract to aerosolized BZ. The chemical protective ensemble protects the skin against contact with BZ or other incapacitating agents dispersed as fine solid particles or in solution. Protection against ingestion would depend upon a high index of suspicion for BZ contaminated food or drink.

MECHANISM OF TOXICITY

BZ may be dispersed as an aerosolized collection of small particles. Alternately, it may be dissolved in a solvent such as DMSO to enhance percutaneous absorption. Bioavailability via ingestion and by inhalation of one-micron particles approximates 80%, and 40 to 50%, respectively, of a parenterally delivered dose of BZ. Percutaneous absorption of BZ dissolved in propylene glycol yields, after a latent period of up to 24 hours, serum levels approximately 5 to 10% of those achieved with IV or intramuscular (IM) administration. Although inhalation of aerosolized BZ is probably the greatest risk on the battlefield, terrorists may choose to disseminate BZ in forms that provide significant opportunities for ingestion and absorption through the skin.

Following absorption, BZ is systemically distributed to most organs and tissues of the body. Its ability to reach synapses and neuromuscular and neuroglandular junctions throughout the body is responsible for its PNS effects, whereas its ability to cross the blood-brain barrier confers upon it the ability to cause CNS effects. Atropine and hyoscyamine both cross the placenta and can be found in small quantities in breast milk; whether this is also true for BZ is unclear.

Metabolism of BZ would be expected to occur primarily in the liver, with elimination of unchanged agent and metabolites chiefly in the urine.

TOXICITY

The characteristic that makes BZ an incapacitating rather than a toxic chemical warfare agent is its high safety ratio. The amount required to produce effects is a thousand or more fold less than a fatal dose of the compound. In terms of Ct products (admittedly a sometimes problematic way of measuring dosage received after aerosol exposure, the ICt_{50} (the Ct product needed to produce incapacitation in 50% of an exposed group) for BZ is 112 mg-min/m^3, whereas the LCt_{50} is estimated to be 200,000 mg·min/m^3.

TOXICODYNAMICS (MECHANISM OF ACTION)

The agent BZ and other anticholinergic glycolates act as competitive inhibitors of the neurotransmitter acetylcholine neurons (1) at postjunctional muscarinic receptors in cardiac and smooth muscle and in exocrine (ducted) glands and (2) at postsynaptic receptors in neurons. As the concentration of BZ at these sites increases, the proportion of receptors available for binding to acetylcholine decreases and the end organ "sees" less acetylcholine. (One way of visualizing this process is to imagine BZ coating the surface of the end organ and preventing acetylcholine from reaching its receptors.) Because BZ has little to no agonist activity with respect to acetylcholine, high concentrations of BZ essentially substitute a "dud" for acetylcholine at these sites and lead to clinical effects reflective of understimulation of end organs.

CLINICAL EFFECTS

Peripheral Effects

- Mydriasis, blurred vision
- Dry mouth, skin
- Initially rapid heart rate; later, normal or slow heart rate
- Possible atropine flush

The PNS effects of BZ are, in general, readily understood as those of understimulation of end organs and are qualitatively similar to those of atropine. Decreased stimulation of eccrine and apocrine sweat glands in the skin results in dry skin (an affected patient can be "dry as a bone") and a reduction in the ability to dissipate heat by evaporative cooling. The skin becomes warm ("hot as a hare") partly from decreased sweating and partly from compensatory cutaneous vasodilatation (the patient becomes "red as a beet," with a so-called atropine flush) as the body attempts to shunt a higher proportion of core-temperature blood as close as possible to the surface of the skin. With decreased heat loss, the core temperature itself rises.

Understimulation of other exocrine glands leads to xerostomia (dry mouth, another way in which the patient is "dry as a bone"), thirst, and decreased secretions from lacrimal, nasal, bronchial, and gastrointestinal glands.

Decreased cholinergic stimulation of pupillary sphincter muscles allows alpha-adrenergically innervated pupillary dilating muscles to act essentially unopposed, resulting in mydriasis. (In fact, the cosmetic effect of mydriasis in women who applied extracts of deadly nightshade topically to their eyes explains the name "belladonna" ["beautiful lady"] given to this plant.) Similar effects on cholinergic ciliary muscles produce paralysis of accommodation. Classically, the patient is described as being as "blind as a bat." Other smooth muscle effects from BZ intoxication include decreased bladder tone and decreased urinary force with possibly severe bladder distention (yet another way in which the patient may be said to be "dry as a bone").

BZ typically raises the heart rate initially, but hours later, depending on the dose of BZ, the heart rate falls to normal or may become slow. Either the peripheral vagal blockade has ceased or the stimulation of the vagal nucleus has occurred.

Neither atropine nor BZ can act directly at the postjunctional nicotinic receptors found in skeletal muscle, but BZ-exposed patients nonetheless exhibit muscle weakness. This weakness, along with incoordination, heightened stretch reflexes, and ataxia, is probably due to the effects of BZ at CNS sites.

The PNS effects of BZ are essentially side effects that are useful in diagnosis, but incidental to the CNS effects for which the incapacitating agents were developed. These CNS effects include a dose-dependent decrease in the level of consciousness, beginning with drowsiness and progressing through sedation to stupor and coma. The patient is often disoriented to time and place. Disturbances in judgment and insight appear. The patient may abandon socially imposed restraints and resort to vulgar and inappropriate behavior. Perceptual clues may no longer be readily interpretable, and the patient is easily distracted and may have memory loss, most notably short-term memory. In the face of these deficits, the patient still tries to make sense of his environment and will not hesitate to make up answers on the spot to questions that confuse him. Speech becomes slurred and often senseless, and loss of inflection produces a flat, monotonous voice. References become concrete and semiautomatic with colloquialisms, clichés, profanity, and perseveration. Handwriting also deteriorates. Semiautomatic behavior may also include disrobing (perhaps partly because of increased body temperature), mumbling, and phantom behaviors such as constant picking, plucking, or grasping motions ("woolgathering" or carphology).

Central Effects

- Disturbances in level of consciousness
- Misperceptions and difficulty in interpretation (delusions, hallucinations)
- Poor judgement and insight (denial of illness)
- Short attention span, distractibility, impaired memory (particularly recent)
- Slurred speech, perseveration
- Disorientation
- Ataxia
- Variability (quiet/restless)

Central nervous system mediated perceptual disturbances in BZ poisoning include both illusions (misidentification of real objects) and hallucinations (the perception of objects or attributes that have no objective reality). (Although the phrase "mad as a hatter" refers to poisoning from mercury formerly used by hatters on felt, it can just as well serve as a reminder of CNS effects from anticholinergics.)

Anticholinergic hallucinations differ from the often vague, ineffable, and often transcendent-appearing hallucinations induced by hallucinogenic indoles such as LSD. Hallucinations from BZ tend to be realistic, distinct, easily identifiable (often commonly encountered objects or persons), and panoramic. They also have the tendency to decrease in size during the course of the intoxication.

Another prominent CNS finding in BZ poisoning is behavioral lability, with patients swinging back and forth between quiet confusion or self-absorption in hallucinations, to frank combativeness. Moreover, as other symptoms begin to resolve, intermittent paranoia may be seen. Automatic behaviors common during resolution include the crawling or climbing motions called "progresso obstinato" in old descriptions of dementia.

BZ produces effects not just in individuals, but also in groups. Sharing of illusions and hallucinations (*folie à deux*, *folie en famille*, and "mass hysteria") is exemplified by two BZ-intoxicated individuals who would take turns smoking an imaginary cigarette clearly visible to both of them but to no one else.

TIME COURSE OF EFFECTS

Clinical effects from ingestion or inhalation of BZ appear after an asymptomatic or latent period that may be as little as 30 minutes, or as long as 20 hours; the usual range is 0.5 to 4 hours, with a mean of 2 hours. However, effects may not appear up to 36 hours after skin exposure to BZ.

Once effects appear, their duration is typically 72 to 96 hours and is dose-dependent. Following an ICt_{50} of BZ, severe effects may last 36 hours, but mild effects may persist for an additional day.

The clinical course from BZ poisoning can be divided into the following four stages:

1. Onset or induction (zero to four hours after exposure), characterized by parasympathetic blockade and mild CNS effects.

2. Second phase (4 to 20 hours after exposure), characterized by stupor with ataxia and hyperthermia.

3. Third phase (20 to 96 hours after exposure), in which full-blown delirium is seen but often fluctuates from moment to moment.

4. Fourth phase, or resolution, characterized by paranoia, deep sleep, reawakening, crawling or climbing automatisms, and eventual reorientation.

DIFFERENTIAL DIAGNOSIS

The differential diagnosis for irrational and confused patients is a long one and includes anxiety reactions as well as intoxication with a variety of agents, to include hallucinogenic indoles (such as LSD), cannabinoids (such as the delta-9-tetrahydrocannabinol in marijuana), lead, barbiturates, and bromides. All of these conditions can lead to restlessness, lightheadedness (with associated vertigo and ataxia), confusion, and erratic behavior with or without vomiting. Clues that specifically point to BZ or a related compound are the combination of anticholinergic PNS effects ("dry as a bone," "hot as a hare," "red as a beet," and "blind as a bat") with the CNS effects ("mad as a hatter") of slurred and monotonous speech, automatic behavior (perseveration, disrobing, and phantom behaviors ["woolgathering"]), and vivid, realistic, describable hallucinations (decreasing in size over time) in a patient slipping into and out of delirium.

SIGNS AND SYMPTOMS	POSSIBLE ETIOLOGY
Restlessness, dizziness, or giddiness; failure to obey orders, confusion, erratic behavior; stumbling or staggering; vomiting.	Anticholinergics (e.g., BZ, indoles (e.g., LSD), cannabinols (e.g., marijuana), anxiety reaction, other intoxications (e.g., alcohol, bromides, barbiturates, lead).
Dryness of mouth, tachycardia at rest, elevated temperature, flushing of face; blurred vision, pupillary dilation; slurred or nonsensical speech; hallucinatory behavior; disrobing; mumbling and picking behavior; stupor and coma.	Anticholinergics
Inappropriate smiling or laughter, irrational fear, distractibility, difficulty expressing self, perceptual distortions; labile increase in pupil size, heart rate, blood pressure. Stomach cramps and vomiting may occur.	Indoles (Schizophrenic psychosis may mimic in some respects.)
Euphoric, relaxed, unconcerned daydreaming attitude, easy laughter; hypotension and dizziness on sudden standing.	Cannabinols
Tremor, clinging or pleading, crying; clear answers, decrease in disturbance with reassurance; history of nervousness or immaturity, phobias.	Anxiety reaction

Atropine intoxication from MARK I autoinjector use in a patient not exposed to nerve agents may create similar PNS effects to those seen in BZ intoxication. However, marked confusion from atropine is not normally seen until a total of six or seven autoinjectors have been given (in a hot, dehydrated, or battle-stressed individual, less atropine would probably suffice). Circumstantial evidence may be helpful in this situation. Heat stroke may also generate hot, dry, and confused or stuporous casualties and needs to be considered in the differential diagnosis. Patients with anxiety reactions are usually oriented to time, place, and person but may be trembling, crying, or otherwise panicked. The classic picture of unconcern or "la belle indifférence" may characterize a patient with a conversion reaction, but these patients are also likely to be oriented and lack the anticholinergic PNS signs of BZ poisoning.

MEDICAL MANAGEMENT

The admonition to protect oneself first may be difficult when dealing with any intoxication involving a latent period, since initially asymptomatic exposure to health care providers may already have occurred during the same time frame in which patients were exposed. Protection of medical staff from already absorbed and systemically distributed BZ in a patient is not needed.

General supportive management of the patient includes decontamination of skin and clothing (ineffective for already absorbed agent but useful in preventing further absorption of any agent still in contact with the patient), confiscation of weapons and related items from the patient, and observation. Physical restraint may be required in moderately to severely affected patients. The greatest risks to the patient's life are (1) injuries from his or her own erratic behavior (or from the behavior of similarly intoxicated patients) and (2) hyperthermia, especially in patients who are in hot or humid environments or are dehydrated from overexertion or insufficient water intake. A severely exposed patient might be comatose with serious cardiac arrhythmias and electrolyte disturbances. Management of heat stress assumes a high priority in these patients. Because of the prolonged time course in BZ poisoning, consideration should always be given to evacuation to a higher echelon of care.

As a competitive inhibitor of acetylcholine, BZ effectively decreases the amount of acetylcholine "seen" by postsynaptic and postjunctional receptors throughout the body. Specific antidotal therapy in BZ poisoning is therefore geared toward raising the concentration of acetylcholine in these synapses and junctions. Any compound that causes a rise in acetylcholine concentration can potentially overcome BZ-induced inhibition and restore normal functioning;

even the nerve agent VX has been shown to be effective when given under carefully controlled conditions. The specific antidote of choice in BZ poisoning is the carbamate anticholinesterase physostigmine (eserine; Antilirium®), which temporarily raises acetylcholine concentrations by binding reversibly to anticholinesterase on the postsynaptic or postjunctional membrane. Physostigmine is similar in many ways to pyridostigmine and is equally effective when used as a pre-exposure antidotal enhancer ("pretreatment") in individuals at high risk for subsequently encountering soman. However, physostigmine is not used for this purpose because the doses required cause vomiting through CNS mechanisms. In the case of BZ poisoning, a nonpolar compound such as physostigmine is used specifically because penetration into the brain is required in those individuals who already have CNS effects from BZ.

In BZ-intoxicated patients, physostigmine is minimally effective during the first four hours after exposure but is very effective after four hours. Oral dosing generally requires one and a half times the amount of antidote as does IM or IV administration. However, effects from a single intramuscular injection of physostigmine last only about 60 minutes, necessitating frequent re-dosing. It must be emphasized that physostigmine does not shorten the clinical course of BZ poisoning and that relapses will occur if treatment is discontinued prematurely. The temptation to substitute a slow IV infusion for intramuscular injections should be tempered by the awareness that IV infusion may lead to nerve-agent-like bradycardia and too rapid infusion might cause arrhythmias, excessive secretions (to the point of compromising air exchange), and convulsions. (See below under Toxicity). Moreover, the sodium bisulfite in commercially available preparations of physostigmine may cause life-threatening allergic responses.

Suggested dosages for physostigmine in the treatment of BZ poisoning follow:

Test dose: If the diagnosis is in doubt, a dose of 1 mg might be given. If a slight improvement occurs, routine dosing should begin.

Routine dosing: Doses of about 45 mcg/kg for adults have been recommended. This might be modified by the response. A mental status examination should be done every hour, and the dose and time interval of dosing should be modified according to whether the mental status is improved or not. As the patient improves, the dose requirement will decrease.

Routes of administration:

IM: 45 mcg/kg in adults (20 mcg/kg in children)

IV: 30 mcg/kg slowly (1 mg/min)

PO: 60 mcg/kg if patient is cooperative (because of bitter taste, consider diluting in juice)

For each route, titrate about every 60 minutes to mental status.

HISTORY AND TOXICITY OF PHYSOSTIGMINE

The antagonism between physostigmine (the elixir of calabar bean) and atropine (tincture of belladonna) was first reported in 1864 by a physician who successfully treated prisoners who had become delirious after drinking tincture of belladonna. Physicians did not notice this report until the 1950s when atropine coma (in which 50 mg or so of atropine were given to certain psychiatric patients) was successfully treated with physostigmine after the "therapeutic benefit" had been attained. Again, this went unnoticed until a controlled study, reported in 1967, indicated that anticholinergic intoxication could be successfully, albeit transiently, reversed by physostigmine.

A recent textbook of emergency medicine statec that physostigmine should be used only as "a last resort." It would seem that when a patient needs "last resort" care, it is the absolute wrong time to administer a potent cholinesterase inhibitor.

The administration of physostigmine by the IV route in a delirious but conscious and otherwise health patient is not without peril. It is sometimes difficult to keep a delirious patient quiet long enough to administer the drug (at 1 mg/min in the marketed solution of 1 mg/ml). Even if administered correctly (very slowly), the heart rate may decline from 110 bpm to 45 bpm over a period of one to two minutes. The difference in the onset of the effects after IM and IV administration of physostigmine is a matter of only several minutes, and since its use is rarely lifesaving, this slight difference in time of response is inconsequential.

Physostigmine is a safe and effective antidote if used properly. In a conscious and delirious patient it will produce very effective but transient reversal of both the peripheral and central effects of cholinergic blocking compounds. Its use by the IV route is not without hazards. It absolutely should NOT be used in a patient with cardiorespiratory compromise, hypoxia, or acid base imbalance with a history of seizure disorders or arrhythmias.

TRIAGE

An **immediate** casualty (possible but unlikely) would be one with cardiorespiratory compromise or severe hyperthermia. Immediate attention to ventilation, hemodynamic status, and temperature control could be life-saving. Because of its dangers in a hypoxic or hemodynamically challenged patient, physostigmine should be considered a second-line management option to be used only if adequate attention can simultaneously be given to temperature and other vital signs.

The **delayed** casualty would present with pronounced or worsening anticholinergic CNS signs. Physostigmine should definitely be considered in this kind of patient.

A **minimal** casualty from a strictly medical standpoint might have mild PNS or CNS anticholinergic effects. Given the time course of BZ intoxication, however, these patients should not be considered able to manage themselves or capable of routine return to duty and should be relieved of their weapons, observed, and, if the holding capacity at the current echelon is exceeded, evacuated.

An **expectant** casualty (also possible but unlikely) would have severe cardiorespiratory compromise in a situation in which treatment or evacuation resources are too limited to allow the necessary attention to be directed to him or her.

RETURN TO DUTY

Given the time course of the intoxication, however, early return to duty is probably not a realistic possibility for the majority of casualties who may require observation and management for several days at the least.

RIOT-CONTROL AGENTS
CS, CN

SUMMARY

Signs and Symptoms: burning and pain on exposed mucous membranes and skin, eye pain and tearing, burning in the nostrils, respiratory discomfort, and tingling of the exposed skin.

Detection: no detector.

Decontamination: **Eyes:** thoroughly flush with water, saline, or similar substance. **Skin:** flush with copious amounts of water, alkaline soap and water, or a mildly alkaline solution (sodium bicarbonate or sodium carbonate). Generally, decontamination is not needed if the wind is brisk. Hypochlorite exacerbates the skin lesion and should not be used.

Immediate management: Usually none is necessary; effects are self-limiting.

OVERVIEW

Riot-control agents, also called irritants, lacrimators, and "tear gas," produce transient discomfort and eye closure to render the recipient temporarily incapable of fighting or resisting. Law enforcement agencies use them for riot control, and military forces use them for training and in combat (see below). They have a high LCt_{50} and a low effective Ct_{50}, and therefore have a high safety ratio. Their major activity is to cause pain, burning, or discomfort on exposed mucous membranes and skin; these effects occur within seconds of exposure but seldom persist more than a few minutes after exposure has ended.

HISTORY/MILITARY RELEVANCE

Paris police used riot-control agents to dispel rioters before World War I, and these compounds were the first chemical agents deployed during that war. French soldiers used them with limited success in small skirmishes. About 30 riot-control agents were developed and used, but their use decreased following the advent of more potent compounds.

After World War I, military and law enforcement agencies used CN for various purposes until CS, a more potent and less toxic compound synthesized by Corson and Stoughton (hence the nomenclature) in

1928, replaced it in about 1959. Today CN is in commercially available devices for self-protection (Mace[R]), but CS is the agent otherwise used. The military forces of most countries use it in training as a confidence builder for the protective mask (the "gas chamber exercise"), and the U.S. used it extensively in Vietnam, primarily for tunnel denial. Worldwide, police forces of many countries, e.g., Ireland, France, Russia, and the U.S., use it for crowd control or during riots.

The U.S. excludes these agents from international treaty provisions. They may be used in military situations by presidential order.

The agents in use today are CS and CN. CA is outmoded, CR is a British agent, and DM is neither used nor stockpiled.

PHYSICOCHEMICAL CHARACTERISTICS

Unlike most agents which are liquids under temperate conditions, riot-control agents are solids with low vapor pressures and are dispersed as fine particles or in solution. Dispersion devices include small, hand-held spray cans, large spray tanks, grenades, and larger weapons.

TOXICODYNAMICS (MECHANISM OF ACTION)

The mechanism of biological activity is less well characterized for riot-control agents than for most other agents. Fortunately, a detailed knowledge of the mechanism of action is not necessary for appropriate medical management.

CS and CN are SN_2 alkylating agents (mustard, in contrast, is an SN_1 alkylator) and react readily at nucleophilic sites. Prime targets include sulfhydryl-containing enzymes such as lactic dehydrogenase. In particular, CS reacts rapidly with the disulfhydryl form of lipoic acid, a coenzyme in the pyruvate decarboxylase system. It has been suggested that tissue injury may be related to inactivation of certain of these enzyme systems.

Pain can occur without tissue injury and may be bradykinin mediated. CS causes bradykinin release in vivo and in vitro, and elimination of bradykininogen in vivo abolishes the systemic response to CS.

The initial response to aerosolized CS is an increase in blood pressure and irregular respiration, suggestive of the Sherrington pseudoaffective response. Bypassing the pain receptors of the nose and upper airway by endotracheal administration of CS leads to the same decrease in blood pressure and in respiration seen after intravenous injection. This suggests that the initial pressor effect and irregular respiration are responses to a noxious stimulus rather than pharmacological effects of CS.

CLINICAL EFFECTS

The main effects of riot-control agents are pain, burning, and irritation of exposed mucous membranes and skin. These effects do not differ appreciably from one agent to another except in the case of DM, which will be discussed in a separate section.

Eyes. The eye is the organ most sensitive to riot-control agents. Contact with agent produces a sensation of conjunctival and corneal burning and leads to tearing, blepharospasm, and conjunctival injection. The severe blepharospasm causes the lids to close tightly and produces transient "blindness," an effect that could inhibit the recipient's ability to fight or resist. However, if the recipient opens his eyes, his vision is near normal even if a significant concentration of the agent persists.

Because these compounds are solids, it is possible for a particle or clump to become embedded in the cornea or conjunctiva to cause tissue damage. With the caveat noted below, there is no evidence that this complication has ever occurred; however, a recipient seeking medical care for eye pain after exposure should have his eyes thoroughly decontaminated and undergo thorough ophthalmic examination. It could be necessary to pick out the particles of agent from tissue.

Reviewers examined the evidence for permanent eye damage from riot-control agents. In each instance, the damage was from a weapon fired from close range (about 50% were self-inflicted). The reviewers concluded that the blast force driving the agent deep into tissue (with or without the wadding of the weapon) was the major cause of permanent injuries. This should not happen under normal use.

Nose and mouth. Contact with the delicate mucous membranes of the nose produces a burning sensation, rhinorrhea, and sneezing; a similar burning sensation accompanied by increased salivation occurs after contact with the mouth.

Airways. Inhalation causes burning and irritation of the airways with bronchorrhea, coughing, and a perception of a "tight chest" or an inability to breathe. However, pulmonary function studies done immediately after exposure have shown minimal alterations.

An inhaled irritating compound might be expected to exacerbate a chronic pulmonary disease such as asthma, emphysema, or bronchitis, but this appears not to happen after CS or CN, even though these agents have been used widely in mixed populations. The medical care provider should nevertheless anticipate airway problems in individuals with lung disease, particularly if they are exposed to higher than the average field use concentrations.

There is no evidence that CS causes permanent lung damage after one or several exposures to field concentrations. Following inhalation of lethal amounts, animals died from severe airway damage 12 to 24 hours post-exposure, but survivors from large exposures had minimal or no pulmonary abnormalities. After multiple (50 or more) daily exposures to smaller amounts, animals developed laryngitis and tracheitis.

Skin. Contact with the skin causes a tingling or burning sensation and may cause erythema, particularly if the skin is raw or freshly abraded (e.g., shortly after shaving). The erythema begins several minutes after exposure and generally subsides 45 to 60 minutes after termination of exposure.

Under conditions of high temperature, high humidity, and high concentration of agent, there may be more severe dermatitis starting with erythema hours after exposure and followed by vesication. Generally these are second-degree burns not unlike, but more severe than sunburn. Firemen who entered contaminated buildings after summer riots several decades ago developed these lesions. After stirring up the contaminating particles, they later developed erythema and blisters on their exposed skin.

Hypersensitivity may develop. In one instance, an individual developed generalized vesication and high fever after an uneventful exposure to CS more than 20 years after his only and equally uneventful previous exposure.

Gastrointestinal tract. Gastrointestinal effects usually do not occur with most riot-control agents (DM is an exception), although there may be retching or vomiting if the agent concentration is high, exposure is prolonged, or the individual is sensitive.

Cardiovascular**.** A transient increase in heart rate and blood pressure has occurred in people immediately prior to an exposure to a riot-control agent or immediately after onset of exposure. The heart rate and blood pressure returned essentially to pre-test ranges while exposure continued and may have been caused by the anxiety or the initial pain rather than to a pharmacological effect of these agents. This "alarm reaction" may cause adverse effects in one with pre-existing cardiovascular disease.

Oral ingestion**.** Children occasionally eat CS, and several adults have swallowed CS pellets. Aside from bouts of diarrhea and abdominal cramps (which might have been from the cathartics and antacids used as therapy), their courses have been uneventful. In animals, the LD_{50} is about 200 mg/kg (which is about 14 grams/70-kg person), an amount unlikely to be ingested, even deliberately. A few animals fed lethal amounts (or greater) had gastric irritation or erosions, and several had signs of intestinal perforation. Recommended therapy after ingestion consists of cathartics, antacids, and surgical observation.

Lethality. CN, occasionally in combination with DM, has caused deaths in people who refused to exit a confined space. In each case the agent was used in excess. Death generally occurred hours after initial exposure, and post-mortem findings were those of severe airway damage similar to that seen in animals.

Metabolism. Animals given lethal amounts of CS by intravenous or intraperitoneal administration developed increased blood thiocyanate concentrations hours later, indicating that the malononitrile portion of CS had been metabolized to cyanide. Cyanide was not a factor in causing death (lung damage was). A significant increase in blood concentration of thiocyanate has not been noted after aerosol administration of CS. Several popular databases mention this cyanogenic potential of CS and suggest that treatment of a CS casualty might require therapy for cyanide poisoning (this recommendation is apparently based on the IV or IP administration data). After receiving lethal amounts of CS by inhalation, animals died 12 to 24 hours later from severe airway damage; cyanide was not implicated in their deaths.

ADAMSITE (DM)

The effects of usual field concentrations of DM are similar to those of the other riot-control agents, except that DM has little irritancy to the skin. However, at higher concentrations, DM causes nausea, vomiting, and a feeling of generalized malaise. For this reason, it is called a vomiting agent.

TIME COURSE OF EFFECTS

Except for those produced by DM, the biological effects from these agents begin seconds after exposure and continue for 15 minutes or so after one exits the contamination to fresh, clean air. The effects from DM begin two to four minutes after the onset of exposure and may last an hour or two. (This is advantageous militarily, as an individual unaware of the agent will continue to inhale it for several minutes and absorb a larger dose. He may then vomit, requiring mask removal, which leads to continued inhalation of agent.)

DIFFERENTIAL DIAGNOSIS

Usually the circumstances of exposure make the diagnosis obvious. The history and the few physical signs (conjunctival injection with normal pupils, tearing, etc.) are usually adequate. On a battlefield, the sudden onset of burning pain and irritation might lead one to consider Lewisite or phosgene oxime exposure, but the signs and symptoms of riot-control agents gradually recede, whereas those from the vesicants worsen.

LABORATORY FINDINGS

There are no specific laboratory tests that will confirm the diagnosis. Complications, e.g., infection of a skin lesion, will produce the laboratory findings characteristic of the complication.

MEDICAL MANAGEMENT

The effects of exposure to these agents under the usual field conditions generally are self-limiting and require no specific therapy. Most will disappear in 15 to 30 minutes, although erythema may persist for an hour or longer.

The following section discusses potential complications occurring only under exceptional circumstances, such as exposure to a very large amount of agent (as in an enclosed space), exposure in adverse weather, or experimental studies in humans or animals. They are not to be expected with normal use of these agents.

Less than 1% of exposed people will have effects severe or prolonged enough to cause them to seek medical care. Those who do probably will have eye, airway, or skin complaints. Because there is no antidote for these agents, treatment consists of symptomatic management.

Eyes. The eye should be carefully flushed with water or saline, and impacted particles should be sought. General care consists of a topical solution (many are available) to relieve the irritation and topical antibiotics. An ophthalmologist should be consulted for further evaluation and care.

Pulmonary. These agents may exacerbate chronic disease or unmask latent disease (although there is little evidence of this). Bronchospasm with wheezing and mild distress continuing hours after exposure may occur in a latent asthmatic. More severe effects and respiratory distress may occur in one with chronic bronchitis or emphysema. Management includes oxygen administration (with assisted ventilation, if necessary), bronchodilators if bronchospasm is present, and specific antibiotics dictated by the results of sputum studies (Gram stains of smears followed by culture). A specialist skilled in the treatment of inhalation injury should be consulted early. Animal studies and very limited human data indicate that maximal effects occur 12 hours after exposure.

Skin. The early erythema requires reassurance, but no specific therapy unless severe and prolonged more than an hour or two. The later onset erythema precipitated by a larger exposure in a hot and humid atmosphere is usually more severe and less likely to resolve quickly. It may require the use of soothing compounds such as calamine, camphor, and mentholated creams. Small vesicles should be left intact, but larger ones will ultimately break and should be drained. Irrigation of denuded areas several times a day should be followed by the application of a topical antibiotic. Large, oozing areas have responded to compresses containing substances such as colloidal oatmeal, Burrow's solution, and other dermatologic preparations.

TRIAGE

A person exposed to the usual field concentrations of riot-control agents will probably not be seen at a triage area. Those presenting with complications should be triaged according to the nature of their injuries.

RETURN TO DUTY

Because the effects of field concentrations clear within minutes, the casualty should be returned to duty as soon as possible. Casualties with complications may require evacuation and further medical treatment before returning to duty.

DECONTAMINATION

OVERVIEW

Decontamination is the reduction or removal of chemical agents. Decontamination may be accomplished by removal of these agents by physical means or by chemical neutralization or detoxification. Decontamination of skin is the primary concern, but decontamination of eyes and wounds must also be done when necessary. Personal decontamination is decontamination of self; casualty decontamination refers to the decontamination of casualties; and personnel decontamination usually refers to decontamination of noncasualties.

The most important and most effective decontamination of any chemical exposure is that decontamination done within the first minute or two after exposure. This is self-decontamination, and this early action by the soldier will make the difference between survival (minimal injury) and death (severe injury). Good training can save lives.

Decontamination of casualties is an enormous task. The process requires dedication of both large numbers of personnel and large amounts of time. Even with appropriate planning and training, the requirement demands a significant contribution of resources.

Liquids and solids are the only substances that can be effectively removed from the skin. It is generally not possible or necessary to decontaminate vapor. Removal from the atmosphere containing the vapor is all that is required.

Many substances have been evaluated for their usefulness in skin decontamination.

The most common problems with potential decontaminants are irritation of the skin, toxicity, ineffectiveness, or high cost. An ideal decontaminant will rapidly and completely decontaminate all known chemical and biological warfare agents. Furthermore, a suitable skin decontaminant must have certain properties that are not requirements for decontaminants for equipment. Recognized desirable traits of a skin decontaminant include the following:

- Neutralization of all agents

- Safety (compound to be both nontoxic and noncorrosive)

- Ease of application by hand

- Readily available

- Rapid action
- Nonproduction of toxic end products
- Stability in long-term storage
- Short-term stability (after issue to unit/individual)
- Affordability
- Nonenhancement of percutaneous agent absorption
- No irritability
- Hypoallergenicity
- Ease of disposal

Decontamination issues have been explored since the beginning of modern chemical warfare. After years of research worldwide, simple principles that consistently produce good results still apply.

The first, without equal, is timely physical removal of the agent. To remove the substance by the best means available is the primary objective. Chemical destruction (detoxification) of the offending agent is a desirable secondary objective. Physical removal is imperative because none of the chemical means of destroying these agents do so instantaneously. While decontamination preparations such as fresh hypochlorite react rapidly with some agents (e.g., the half time for destruction of VX by hypochlorite at a pH of 10 is 1.5 minutes), the half times of destruction of other agents, such as mustard, are much longer. If a large amount of agent is present initially, a longer time is needed to completely neutralize the agent to a harmless substance.

Decontamination studies have been conducted using common household products. The goal of these studies was identification of decontaminants for civilians, as well as field expedients for the soldier. Timely use of water, soap and water, or flour, followed by wet tissue wipes, produced results equal, nearly equal, or in some instances, better than those produced by the use of Fuller's Earth, Dutch Powder, and other compounds. (Fuller's Earth and Dutch Powder are decontamination agents currently fielded by some European countries.) This is easily understood because (1) no topical decontaminant has ever shown efficacy with penetrated agent, (2) agents in large enough quantity, especially vesicants, may begin penetrating the skin before complete reactive decontamination (detoxification) takes place, and (3) early physical removal is most important.

Military personnel may be questioned for guidance by local civilian authorities or may deal with supply shortages in the field. Knowledge of the U.S.' doctrinal solutions may not suffice in these situations, and awareness of alternative methods of decontamination will prove very beneficial.

However, it is not so much what method is used, rather it is how and when it is used. Chemical agents should be removed as quickly and completely as possible by the best means available.

The M291 resin kit and 0.5% hypochlorite for casualty decontamination are state-of-the-art. The M291 Kit is new, whereas hypochlorite has been around since World War I. The M291 Kit is the best universal dry decontaminant for skin. Fresh 0.5% hypochlorite solution with an alkaline pH is the best available universal liquid decontaminating agent. Liquids are best for large or irregular surface areas. Hypochlorite solutions are well suited for medical treatment facilities with adequate water supplies. For hypochlorite to be the best universal liquid skin decontaminant, it has to be relatively fresh (made daily or more frequently, particularly in a warm environment where evaporation will occur) and at a concentration of 0.5% at an alkaline pH. Hypochlorite solutions are for use on skin and soft tissue wounds only. Hypochlorite should not be used in abdominal wounds, open chest wounds, on nervous tissue, or in the eye. Surgical irrigation solutions should be used in liberal amounts in the abdomen and chest. All such solutions should be removed by suction instead of sponging and wiping. Only copious amounts of water, normal saline, or eye solutions are recommended for the eye. Contaminated wounds will be discussed later.

The M291 resin kit is best for spot decontamination of skin only. It rapidly adsorbs the chemical agent with carbonaceous material, physically removing the agent from skin contact. Later, an ion exchange resin neutralizes the offending agent by chemical detoxification. Since the M291 Kit is small and dry and easily carried by the soldier, it is well suited for field use. It will be the early intervention with the use of this kit that will reduce chemical injury and save lives in most cases. Decontamination of the casualty using an M291 Kit does not obviate the need for decontamination at a field facility. The decontamination station is more conducive to thorough decontamination. Chemical agent transfer is a potential problem that can be resolved by a second deliberate decontamination. Decontamination at the medical treatment facility prevents spread of the agent to areas of the body previously uncontaminated, contamination of personnel assisting the patient, and contamination of the medical facility.

CERTIFICATION OF DECONTAMINATION

Certification of decontamination is accomplished by any of the following: processing through the decontamination facility; M-8 paper; M-9 tape; M256A1 ticket; or by the CAM (Chemical Agent Monitor). If proper procedure is followed, the possibility of admitting a contaminated casualty to a field medical facility is extremely small. The probability of admitting a dangerously contaminated casualty is minuscule to nonexistent. Fear is the worst enemy, not the contaminated soldier.

METHODS OF DECONTAMINATION

Three basic methods of decontamination are physical removal, chemical deactivation, and biological deactivation of the agent. Biological deactivation has not been developed to the point of being practical.

PHYSICAL REMOVAL

Several types of physical and chemical methods are at least potentially suitable for decontaminating equipment and material. Flushing or flooding contaminated skin or material with water or aqueous solutions can remove or dilute significant amounts of agent. Scraping with a wooden stick, i.e., a tongue depressor or Popsicle stick, can remove bulk agent by physical means. For the decontamination of clothing only, adsorbents and containment materials (to be used on outer garments before their removal and disposal) have been considered. A significant advantage of most physical methods is their nonspecificity. Since they work nearly equally well on chemical agents regardless of chemical structure, knowledge of the specific contaminating agent(s) is not required.

Flushing with Water or Aqueous Solutions. When animal skin contaminated with GB was flushed with water (a method in which physical removal predominates over hydrolysis of the agent), 10.6 times more GB was required to produce the same mortality rate as when no decontamination occurred. In another study, the use of water alone produced better results than high concentrations of hypochlorite (i.e., 5.0% or greater, which are not recommended for skin). Timely, copious flushing with water physically removes the agent and will produce good results.

Adsorbent Materials. Adsorption refers to the formation and maintenance of a condensed layer of a substance, such as a chemical agent, on the surface of a decontaminant as illustrated by the adsorption of gases by charcoal particles and by the decontaminants described in this section. Some NATO nations use adsorbent decontaminants in an attempt to reduce the quantity of chemical agent available for uptake through the skin. In emergency situations, dry powders such as soap detergents, earth, and flour, may be useful. Flour, followed by wiping with wet tissue paper, is reported to be effective against GD, VX, and HD.

M291 Resin. The current method of battlefield decontamination by the individual soldier involves the use of a carbonaceous adsorbent, a polystyrene polymeric, and ion exchange resins (M291). The resultant black resin is both reactive and adsorbent. The M291 Kit has been extensively tested and proven highly effective for skin decontamination. It consists of a wallet-like carrying pouch containing six individual decontamination packets. Each packet contains a nonwoven, fiberfill-laminated pad impregnated with the decontamination compounds. Each pad provides the individual with a single step, nontoxic/nonirritating decontamination application that can be used on the skin, including the face, and around wounds. Instructions for use are marked on the case and packets. The individual decontamination pads are impregnated with the decontamination compound, "Ambergard XE-555 Resin", which is the black, free-flowing, resin-based powder. As the pad is scrubbed over the contaminated skin, the chemicals are rapidly transferred into and trapped in the interior of the resin particles. The presence of acidic and basic groups in the resin promotes the destruction of trapped chemical agents by acid and base hydrolysis. Because the resin is black, it maps out the areas that have been decontaminated.

CHEMICAL METHODS

Three types of chemical mechanisms have been used for decontamination: water/soap wash, oxidation, and acid/base hydrolysis.

Mustard (HD) and the persistent nerve agent VX contain sulfur molecules that are readily subject to oxidation reactions. VX and the other nerve agents (GA, GB, GD, and GF) contain phosphorus groups that can be hydrolyzed. Therefore, most chemical decontaminants are designed to oxidize HD and VX and to hydrolyze nerve agents (VX and the G series).

Water/Soap Wash. Both fresh water and sea water have the capacity to remove chemical agents not only through mechanical force, but also via slow hydrolysis; however, the generally low solubility and slow rate of diffusion of chemical warfare agents in water significantly limit the agent hydrolysis rate.

The predominant effect of water and water/soap solutions is the physical removal or dilution of agents; however, slow hydrolysis does occur particularly with alkaline soaps. In the absence of hypochlorite solutions or other appropriate means of removing chemical agents, these methods are considered reasonable options.

Oxidation/Hydrolysis. The most important category of chemical decontamination reactions is oxidative chlorination. This term covers the "active chlorine" chemicals like hypochlorite. The pH of a solution is important in determining the amount of active chlorine concentration. An alkaline solution is advantageous. Hypochlorite solutions act universally against the organophosphorus and mustard agents.

Both VX and HD contain sulfur atoms that are readily subject to oxidation. Current doctrine specifies the use of a 0.5% sodium or calcium hypochlorite solution for decontamination of skin and a 5% solution for equipment.

Hydrolysis. Chemical hydrolysis reactions are of two types, acid and alkaline. Acid hydrolysis is of negligible importance for agent decontamination because the hydrolysis rate of most chemical agents is slow, and adequate acid catalysis is rarely observed. Alkaline hydrolysis is initiated by the nucleophilic attack of the hydroxide ion on the phosphorus atoms found in VX and the G agents. The hydrolysis rate is dependent on the chemical structure and reaction conditions such as pH, temperature, the kind of solvent used, and the presence of catalytic reagents. The rate increases sharply at pH values higher than 8 and increases by a factor of 4 for every 10°C rise in temperature. Several of the hydrolytic chemicals are effective in detoxifying chemical warfare agents; unfortunately, many of these (e.g., NaOH) are unacceptably damaging to the skin. Alkaline pH hypochlorite hydrolyzes VX and the G agents quite well.

WOUND DECONTAMINATION

All casualties entering a medical unit after experiencing a chemical attack are to be considered contaminated unless there is certification of non-contamination. The initial management of a casualty contaminated by chemical agents will require removal of MOPP and decontamination with 0.5% hypochlorite before treatment within the field treatment facility.

Initial decontamination. During initial decontamination in the decontamination areas, bandages are removed and the wounds are flushed; the bandages are replaced only if bleeding recurs. Tourniquets are replaced with clean tourniquets and the sites of the original tourniquets decontaminated. Splints are thoroughly decontaminated, but removed only by a physician.

The new dressings are removed in the operating room and submerged in a 5% solution of hypochlorite or placed in a plastic bag and sealed.

General considerations. Of the agents discussed, only two types, the vesicants and nerve agents, might present a hazard from wound contamination. Cyanide is quite volatile, so it is extremely unlikely that liquid cyanide will remain in a wound, and it requires a very large amount of liquid cyanide to produce vapor adequate to cause effects.

Mustard converts to a cyclic compound within minutes of absorption into a biological milieu, and the cyclic compound rapidly (minutes) reacts with blood and tissue components. These reactions will take place with the components of the wound--the blood, the necrotic tissue, and the remaining viable tissue. If the amount of bleeding and tissue damage is small, mustard will rapidly enter the surrounding viable tissue where it will quickly biotransform and attach to tissue components (and its biological behavior will be much like an intramuscular absorption of the agent).

Although nerve agents cause their toxic effects by their very rapid attachment to the enzyme acetylcholinesterase, they also quickly react with other enzymes and tissue components. As they do with mustard, the blood and necrotic tissue of the wound will "buffer" nerve agents. Nerve agent that reaches viable tissue will be rapidly absorbed, and since the toxicity of nerve agents is quite high (a lethal amount is a small drop), it is unlikely that casualties who have had much nerve agent in a wound will survive to reach medical care.

Potential risk to the surgeon from possibly contaminated wounds arises from agent on foreign bodies in the wound and from thickened agents.

Thickened agents. Thickened agents are chemical agents that have been mixed with another substance (commonly an acrylate) to increase their persistency. They are not dissolved as quickly in biological fluids, nor are they absorbed by tissue as rapidly as other agents. VX, although not a thickened agent, is absorbed less quickly than other nerve agents and may persist in the wound longer than other nerve agents.

Thickened agents in wounds require more precautions. Casualties with thickened nerve agents in wounds are unlikely to survive to reach surgery. Thickened HD has delayed systemic toxicity and can persist in wounds even when the large fragments of cloth have been removed. Though the vapor hazard to surgical personnel is extremely low, contact hazard from thickened agents does remain and should always be assumed.

No country is currently known to stockpile thickened agents. In a chemical attack, the intelligence and chemical staffs should be able to identify thickened agents and to alert medical personnel of their use.

Off-gassing. The risk from vapor off-gassing from chemically contaminated shrapnel and cloth in wounds is very low and not significant. Further, there is no vapor release from contaminated wounds without foreign bodies. Off-gassing from a wound during surgical exploration will be negligible (or zero). No eye injury will result from off-gassing from any of the agents. A chemical-protective mask is not required for surgical personnel.

Foreign material. The contamination of wounds with mustard or nerve agents is basically confined to the foreign material (e.g., battle dress uniform (BDU) and protective garment in the wound). The removal of this cloth from the wound effectively eliminates the hazard. There is little chemical risk associated with individual fibers left in the wound. No further decontamination of the wound for chemical agent is necessary.

Wound contamination assessment. The CAM can be used to assist in locating contaminated objects within a wound; however, 30 seconds are required to achieve a bar reading. The CAM detects vapor, but may not detect liquid (a thickened agent or liquid on a foreign body) deep within a wound. A single bar reading on CAM with the inlet a few millimeters from the wound surface indicates that a vapor hazard does not exist.

Hypochlorite. Diluted hypochlorite (0.5%) is an effective skin decontaminant for patient use. The solution should be made up fresh daily with a pH in the alkaline range. Plastic bottles containing 6 ounces of calcium hypochlorite are currently fielded for this purpose.

Hypochlorite solution is contraindicated for the eye. This substance may result in corneal opacities. It is also not recommended for brain and spinal cord injuries. Irrigation of the abdomen may lead to adhesions and is therefore also contraindicated. The use of hypochlorite in the thoracic cavity may be less of a problem, but the hazard is still unknown.

Wound exploration/debridement. Surgeons and assistants are advised to wear a pair of well-fitting (thin), butyl rubber gloves or double latex surgical gloves and to change them often until they are certain there are no foreign bodies or thickened agents in the wound. This is especially important where puncture is likely because of the presence of bone spicules or metal fragments.

The wound should be explored with surgical instruments rather than with fingers. Pieces of cloth and associated debris must not be examined closely, but quickly disposed of in a container of 5% hypochlorite. The wound can then be checked with the CAM, which may direct the surgeon to further retained material. It takes about 30 seconds to get a stable reading from the CAM. A rapid pass over the wound will not detect remaining contamination. The wound is debrided and excised as normal, maintaining a no-touch technique. Removed fragments of tissue are dropped into hypochlorite. Bulky tissue such as an amputated limb should be placed in a plastic or rubber bag (chemical proof) which is then sealed.

Hypochlorite solution (0.5%) may be instilled into deep, noncavity wounds following the removal of contaminated cloth. This solution should be removed by suction to an appropriate disposal container. Within a short time, i.e., five minutes, this contaminated solution will be neutralized and nonhazardous. Subsequent irrigation with saline or other surgical solutions should be performed.

Penetrating abdominal wounds caused by large fragments or containing large pieces of chemically contaminated cloth will be uncommon. Surgical practices should be effective for the majority of wounds in identifying and removing the focus of remaining agent within the peritoneum. When possible, the CAM may be used to assist. Saline, hydrogen peroxide, or other irrigating solutions do not necessarily decontaminate agents, but may dislodge material for recovery by aspiration with a large bore sucker. The irrigation solution should not be swabbed out manually with surgical sponges. The risk to patients and medical attendants is minuscule. However, safe practice suggests that any irrigation solution should be considered potentially contaminated. Following aspiration by suction, the suction apparatus and the solution should be disposed of in a solution of 5% hypochlorite.

Superficial wounds should be subjected to thorough wiping with 0.5% hypochlorite and subsequent irrigation with normal saline.

Instruments that have come into contact with possible contamination should be placed in 5% hypochlorite for ten minutes prior to normal cleansing and sterilization. Reusable linen should be checked with the CAM, M-8 paper, or M-9 tape for contamination. If found to be contaminated, it should be disposed of in a 5 to 10% hypochlorite solution.

CONCLUSIONS

Decontamination at the medical treatment facility is directed toward: (1) eliminating any agent transferred to the patient during removal of protective clothing; (2) decontaminating or containing of contaminated clothing and personal equipment; and (3) maintaining an uncontaminated treatment facility.

Current doctrine specifies the use of 0.5% hypochlorite solution or the M291 Kit for contaminated skin. These are both state-of-the-art decontamination preparations, one old, and one new.

Fabric and other foreign bodies that have been introduced into a wound have the capacity to sequester and slowly release chemical agent presenting a liquid hazard to both the patient and medical treatment personnel. There is no vapor hazard to surgical personnel. Protective masks are not necessary.

CASUALTY MANAGEMENT IN A CONTAMINATED AREA

OVERVIEW

In a contaminated environment, casualties enter a medical treatment facility through the contaminated casualty receiving area. This occurs at all echelons of medical care that are at risk for receiving contaminated casualties. The purpose of this area is to provide for the removal of all chemical contamination from the casualty before he enters the clean medical treatment facility, and as a result, to maintain a contamination free treatment area where maximal medical care can be provided.

The components of this receiving area are as follows:

- arrival point
- triage area
- emergency treatment area
- decontamination area(s)
- "hot line"

After crossing the hot line, the casualty enters the clean treatment area and, after treatment, enters the clean disposition area. There are two disposition areas. One is for clean casualties (decontaminated patients from the clean treatment area). The other is for "dirty" casualties, casualties who were not decontaminated because they did not need treatment at this echelon. The latter casualties will come from the triage area and the contaminated emergency treatment area.

The exact function and staffing and other support of each of these areas will depend on the size of the medical facility. At a Battalion Aid Station (BAS), for example, staffing is limited, and the same senior medical NCO will usually be both the triage officer and the emergency treatment care provider. The decontamination areas will be staffed by a limited number of augmented personnel, and very limited medical care can be provided in the clean treatment area. At a higher echelon of medical care, another type of medical professional will be the triage officer, a second medical professional, the emergency care provider, and if augmented personnel are not plentiful, the decontamination team might be supplemented by nonmedical personnel from the hospital staff.

The following is intended as an introduction to each of these stations. Detailed information can be found elsewhere (Appendix).

ARRIVAL POINT

The arrival point is the entrance to the casualty receiving area. There should be one clearly marked road for incoming traffic and another clearly marked road for outgoing traffic. Ambulatory casualties will use the same routes. From this area ambulatory casualties will walk to the triage area, and litter bearers will carry litter patients to the triage area.

TRIAGE AREA

In this area the triage officer will quickly evaluate each casualty and place him into one of the triage categories, immediate, minimal, delayed, or expectant. The triage officer might be a senior medic in a BAS and a physician or physician's assistant in larger medical units. His ability to evaluate the casualty will be limited because both he and the casualty will be in MOPP IV.

Those casualties needing immediate care will be sent to the emergency treatment station (also in the contaminated area). Casualties classified as minimal might also be sent to this area, if the appropriate care can be provided in a contaminated environment. The purpose of this is to return them to duty quickly and to lessen the workload on the decontamination teams. However, the types of injuries that can be treated without breaking the integrity of the protective garment are small, and once the integrity of the protective garment is violated, the casualty will need a new protective garment. He might go through decontamination to don his second battle dress overgarment (BDO) in the clean area of that facility, or he will be returned to his unit for reissue of a BDO, in which case he will bypass the decontamination area at his current echelon. (Administration of MARK I Kits is an example of treatment that can be given without breaking the seal of the protective garment; however, if the casualty is ambulatory, the administration of MARK I Kits is self or buddy-aid.) Those casualties classified as delayed will be sent to a decontamination area if they require care in the clean treatment area, or to the contaminated disposition area for evacuation without on-site treatment (bypassing the decontamination area). The expectant casualty will be temporarily set aside for later re-evaluation.

EMERGENCY TREATMENT AREA

In a BAS, the same senior medic who triages might also provide emergency treatment. At larger field treatment facilities, the triage and emergency treatment areas will be separate with different staffs.

The emergency treatment care provider provides assistance to the immediate and minimal casualties.

The care that can be provided in this area is limited because both the casualty and care provider are completely enclosed in protective garments, and the time the single care provider can allocate to a single patient is limited. To some extent, care is limited because this is a contaminated area, but this limitation is relative, not absolute. This area is downwind of the clean area; the only vapor hazard is vapor from liquid that enters the area on the contaminated garments of patients. The amount of vapor arising from this small amount of liquid should be minuscule, and it will quickly dissipate in a breeze. Ventilation of a newly apneic patient will be limited more by the lack of personnel to squeeze the Ambu bag than by the risk of forcing more chemical vapor into the casualty's lungs. Intravenous injections can be given and intravenous fluids can be started after thorough decontamination of the skin site and the care provider's gloves. Minor suturing can be done in this area using the same precautions. The time needed by the single medical care provider to perform these procedures is probably the limiting consideration, not the risk of further contamination.

However, any care or injury that violates the protective garment will necessitate reissue of the garment, and before reissue, the casualty must be decontaminated at this or a rear echelon. At a BAS, for example, once any part of the protective garment is compromised, the casualty who is otherwise able to return to duty must be supplied with new garments. He might go through the decontamination procedure at his current echelon to don his own second BDO in the clean area, or he might be evacuated without decontamination (in a dirty vehicle) for supply at his unit.

In some circumstances, an additional task of the medical care provider at this station will be to irrigate or decontaminate a wound and surrounding area to wash out or decontaminate any remaining agent or exposed areas of skin that seem to be the site of agent exposure. A symptomatic casualty exposed to nerve agent in a wound or on unprotected skin might present at a medical facility while still absorbing agent from the wound or skin surface. It is unlikely that there will be active agent in a wound (unless a foreign body is present), but it is good practice to flush the site. Immediate decontamination will remove this source of further exposure. Because of the latent period from mustard exposure, when a mustard casualty presents for treatment, it is unlikely that immediate decontamination of the exposure site will benefit him. It is equally unlikely that active agent will be present on skin or in a wound (although he needs to be routinely decontaminated before he enters the clean treatment area). Amounts of a decontamination solution suitable for flushing sites of potential contamination should be among the equipment at the emergency treatment station.

After treating the casualty, the emergency treatment provider will send the casualty (1) back to duty (if there has been no violation of his protective encapsulation), (2) to the contaminated disposition area, bypassing the decontamination procedure and clean treatment facility, or (3) to the decontamination area. Casualties who would be sent to the contaminated disposition area (for "dirty" evacuation) are those who need treatment (or hospitalization) later, but do not need immediate care, and those who need supply at their unit. These will be evacuated in the contaminated evacuation vehicle. Those who will be sent to the decontamination area are casualties who need immediate treatment in the clean treatment area and can don their own second BDO in the clean area. For reasons noted below, before he is sent for decontamination, a casualty must be stabilized so that he can survive 20 to 30 minutes without further care.

DECONTAMINATION AREAS

There are two decontamination areas, one for litter casualties and one for ambulatory casualties. The relative use of each area will probably differ from one echelon of medical care to another. For example, at the BAS stable litter, casualties with nonprogressing injuries (a delayed casualty) will bypass decontamination and be sent directly to the contaminated evacuation area. At higher echelons of care with the capability to care for these casualties, all litter patients will be decontaminated. At the BAS, attempts will be made to treat walking casualties and return them to duty.

Decontamination is time and labor intensive. Estimates of the time required to decontaminate a litter patient range from 8 to 20 minutes. A medic supervises the litter decontamination area, but he can provide little or no medical care during this procedure. He cannot support ventilation, nor can he assist a suddenly apneic casualty.

Personnel performing litter decontamination wear butyl rubber aprons over their protective garments. The ambient temperature and humidity dictate their work-rest cycle, but even under temperate conditions the work period is short, necessitating frequent change of personnel. Three people are needed for litter patient decontamination, although two might suffice if one is strong, as patient lifting is necessary.

Litter Decontamination Area

There are two stations in this area, the clothing removal station and the skin decontamination station.

At the clothing removal station (litter), two people work together, one on each side of the litter, to (in order):

- Decontaminate the mask and hood.

- Remove the hood (but leave mask in place).

- Decontaminate the casualty's mask and area around the mask.

- Remove the field medical card.

- Remove gross contamination from the casualty's protective garment.

- Cut and remove the protective garment jacket.

- Cut and remove the protective garment trousers.

- Remove outer gloves.

- Remove the overboots.

- Remove the combat boots.

- Remove inner clothing and underwear (in the same order and using the same procedures as with the protective garments).

- Check for contamination.

At this time, the nude patient is transferred to the skin decontamination litter using a three-person roll lift.

During clothing removal, the aidman removes tourniquets after placing a new one an inch or so higher and cuts away bandages and irrigates wounds (replacing the bandage only if bleeding recurs). He also thoroughly decontaminates splints, but does not remove them.

On the skin decontamination litter, spot decontamination (only) is done on areas of potential contamination. These include the neck, lower face, and wrists and also areas under breaks in the protective ensemble, including areas around wound sites.

After final monitoring for contamination, the casualty is carried on the litter to the shuffle pit and there is moved to a clean litter provided by a team from the clean side of the hot line. The mask is removed further upwind at the entrance to the clean treatment area.

Ambulatory Decontamination Area

A member of the decontamination team might help the walking patient, or walking patients might help each other to remove their garments. The steps in this procedure are as follows:

- Drop the load-bearing equipment.

- Decontaminate and remove the hood.

- Decontaminate the mask and surrounding skin.

- Place the field medical card in a plastic bag.

- Remove all gross contamination from the overgarment.

- Remove the overgarment jacket.

- Remove the rubber gloves.

- Remove the overboots.

- Remove overgarment trousers.

- Remove cotton glove liners.

- Check the battle dress uniform (BDU) and surrounding skin for contamination (and decontaminate any spots of contamination found).

- Lift the mask (while the casualty has his breath held and eyes closed).

- Wipe the face.

- Replace, seal, and clear the mask.

During this procedure the medic changes tourniquets and removes bandages as described in the previous section. The casualty, dressed in his BDU (including mask), thoroughly dusts his boots as he proceeds through the shuffle pit (the hot line) to the clean treatment area. The mask is removed further upwind at the entrance to the clean treatment area.

If, because of the nature of his wounds, his BDU is removed, the casualty becomes a litter patient.

HOT LINE

The hot line is an arbitrarily established line that demarcates the area of liquid-agent contamination from an area that is liquid-agent free. Once established, it should be clearly marked using engineer tape or another marker to ensure that liquid contamination or a person with potential liquid contamination does not cross into the clean area. This might necessitate the use of concertina wire or armed guards. The only entrance to the clean treatment area is through the decontamination stations.

When the medical facility is set up in a clean area (no liquid contamination), all the ground behind the hot line is clean except the holding area for contaminated casualties waiting to be evacuated and the routes traversed by the contaminated evacuation vehicles. These should be far to the side of the contaminated triage and treatment areas. In other circumstances, the clean treatment area will be an oasis surrounded by the hot line.

CHEMICAL DEFENSE EQUIPMENT

This overview is divided into four sections:

- Individual Protection
- Individual Decontamination
- Detection and Alarms
- Patient Protective Equipment

Listed under each item are the 13-digit stock number for the item and the technical manual (TM) describing the use and maintenance of the item.

Individual Protection

This section includes standard "A" chemical defense equipment (CDE) issued to each soldier, which consists of the following:

- M17A2 Protective Mask
- M24 and M25A1 Protective Masks
- M40 and M42 Protective Masks

- Battle Dress Overgarment

- Chemical Protective Gloves and Overboots

Mask, Chemical-Biological: Field

4240-01-143-2017 - X-Small
4240-01-143-2018 - Small
4240-01-143-2019 - Medium
4240-01-143-2020 - Large

TM 3-4240-279-10
TM 3-4240-279-20&P

The M17A2 protective mask is designed to protect the wearer from field concentrations of all known chemical, biological, and riot-control agents. When worn correctly, the mask will protect the face, eyes, and respiratory tract. Wearing the ABC-M6A2 Hood (4240-00-021-8695) attached to the M17A2 mask further protects the soldier's head, neck, and shoulder areas.

The protective mask contains two M13A2 Filter Elements (4240-00-165-5026). Filtration through these elements involves two separate but complimentary mechanisms: (1) impaction and adsorption of agent molecules onto ASC Whetlerite Carbon filtration media and (2) impaction on a high efficiency particulate air filter paper of particles with an average diameter of 0.3 microns.

Maintenance, and when necessary, replacement of the crucial filter elements, are of the utmost priority. The filters must be replaced whenever any of the following occurs:

- The elements are immersed in water.
- The elements are crushed, cut, or otherwise damaged.
- Excessive breathing resistance is encountered.
- The "ALL CLEAR" signal is given after exposure to AC (hydrogen cyanide) or CK (cyanogen chloride).
- Thirty days elapse in the combat theater of operations (the filters must be replaced every 30 days).
- Supply Bulletin 3-30-2 indicates lot number expiration.
- When ordered by the unit commander.

Two styles of optical inserts for the protective mask are available for soldiers requiring visual correction. The M17 optical insert (6540-01-060-

0611), which has a wire frame, is considered the safer of the two and is more easily fitted into the mask; a prong-type optical insert (6540-00-935-6573) is also available.

Fitting the drinking tube of the mask into the M-1 canteen cap (4240-00-930-2077) allows the wearer to drink while in a chemical environment. However, restriction of fluid intake to water obtained in this manner is likely to lead to dehydration, especially when protective clothing must be worn in a hot environment. Drinking before anticipated donning of the mask must therefore be enforced through the use of command directed drinking.

NOTE: Before the wearer drinks via the M-1 cap and the drinking tube, he must verify by using M8 Chemical Detection Paper that the canteen and coupling half are not contaminated. Task 031-503-1006 STP 21-1-SMCT, October 1990.

Mask, Chemical-Biological: Aircraft, ABC-M24

4240-00-808-8799 - Small
4240-00-776-4384 - Medium
4240-00-808-8798 - Large

Mask, Chemical-Biological: Tank, M25A1

4240-00-994-8751 - Small
4240-00-994-8750 - Medium
4240-00-994-8752 - Large

TM 3-4240-280-10
TM 3-4240-280-20&P

Each of these masks when properly fitted and worn protect the wearer's face, eyes, and respiratory tract from field concentrations of all known chemical, biological, and riot-control agents. The ABC-M7 protective hood (4240-00-021-8695) used with the M24 mask, or the ABC-M5 protective hood (4240-00-860-8987) used with the M25A1 mask will, in addition, protect the head, neck, and shoulders. The aviator draws the M7 hood over his helmet after first donning the M24 mask. Filtered air for each of these masks arrives through a hose attached by a metal connector and coupling to an M10A1 CB canister (4240-00-127-7186) containing the same ASC Whetlerite carbon found in the M13A2 filter elements of the M17A2 mask. The M10A1 CB canister must be changed whenever one of the following occurs:

- The coupling or the connector is bent or heavily rusted.

• The coupling-to-canister connection is not tight.

• The canister has cracks, breaks, or dents over 1/4 inch deep.

• Over 10% of the seams are corroded.

• The canister has been immersed in water.

• Excessive resistance to breathing is encountered.

• Supply Bulletin 3-30-2 indicates lot number expiration.

• Sixty days have elapsed after exposure to a toxic chemical agent.

Only the prong-type of optical insert fits the M24 and M25A1 masks. Neither mask possesses a drinking tube. Wearers must become familiar with the standard procedure detailed in STP 21-1-SMCT, October 1990, Soldier's Manual of Common Tasks, Task #031-503-1006: Drink from Canteen while Wearing Your Protective Mask. Differences between the masks include the following:

• The ABC-M24 mask has an M-8 oxygen supply adapter (4240-00-848-6074) to be used at altitudes requiring oxygen or when using a bailout bottle.

• The M133/U microphone for the M24 mask and the M116G microphone for the M25A1 mask permit use of the on-board intercom system and the vehicle radios, respectively.

• The M17 carrier for the M24 mask is worn on the right side to prevent interference with controls, especially on fixed-wing aircraft; the M13A1 carrier is worn on the left side.

Chemical-Biological Mask: Field M40

4240-01-258-0061 - Small
4240-01-258-0062 - Medium
4240-01-258-0063 - Large

Chemical-Biological Mask: Combat Vehicle M42

4240-01-258-0064 - Small
4240-01-258-0065 - Medium
4240-01-258-0066 - Large

TM 3-4240-300-10
TM 3-4240-300-20&P

When properly fitted and worn, each of these masks will protect the wearer's face, eyes, and respiratory tract from field concentrations of all known chemical, biological, and riot-control agents.

The CB hood (4240-01-260-8723) affords additional protection for the head, neck, and shoulders.

Because both the M40 and M42 masks have drinking tubes positioned around the outlet valve assembly, it is possible to drink water in a chemically contaminated environment. First, the soldier must use M8 paper to verify that the M-1 canteen cap is not contaminated before attaching the drinking tube to the cap. Wearers operating armored vehicles will thus be able to drink water in a contaminated environment.

The only optical insert approved for use in the M40 mask or the M42 mask is a wire-frame type (6540-01-253-8169).

Innovations in these masks include the following:

• Each mask is molded with two voicemitters, one in the front of the mask and one over the cheek. The cheek voicemitter allows the use of the radiotelephone handset without any interference from the protective mask and is interchangeable with the cheek filter canister.

• Each mask uses a NATO standard external filter canister (4240-01-119-2315) of the same type used by both Germany and England. The unit nuclear/biological/chemical (NBC) noncommissioned officer (NCO) may position the canister either on the soldier's right cheek or on his left cheek to allow him to fire the M16A2 rifle from his left or right shoulder, respectively.

• Each protective mask is molded in silicone rubber to allow easy fitting of all wearers, including those who require an extra small M17A2 mask.

• Each mask is made with an in-turned-sealing surface around the entire inner edge of the mask. This allows for a more comfortable seal on the soldier's face.

• The eye lenses in each of these masks are 35% larger than the M17A2 mask eye lens and permit greater range of vision.

Battle Dress Overgarment (BDO)

8415-01-137-1700: XXX-Small
8415-01-137-1701: XX-Small
8415-01-137-1702: X-Small
8415-01-137-1703: Small
8415-01-137-1704: Medium
8415-01-137-1705: Large
8415-01-137-1706: X-Large
8415-01-137-1707: XX-Large

Desert Battle Dress Overgarment (DBDO)
6-Color

8415-01-324-3084: XXX-Small
8415-01-324-3085: XX-Small
8415-01-324-3086: X-Small
8415-01-324-3087: Small
8415-01-324-3088: Medium
8415-01-324-3089: Large
8415-01-324-3090: X-Large
8415-01-324-3091: XX-Large

Desert Battle Dress Overgarment (DBDO)
3-Color

8415-01-327-5346: XXX-Small
8415-01-327-5347: XX-Small
8415-01-327-5348: X-Small
8415-01-327-5349: Small
8415-01-327-5350: Medium
8415-01-327-5351: Large
8415-01-327-5352: X-Large
8415-01-327-5353: XX-Large

The BDO and DBDO have been designed with new features that increase protection in a chemical environment and make wearing the suit less of a heat burden. The suit has more activated charcoal than the previous model, a novel outer cloth weave, and an outer cloth "scotchguard" type treatment resistant to liquid chemical agents. Because of the increased amount of charcoal, the BDO and DBDO can now be worn in an uncontaminated environment for 30 days following removal of the garment from its vapor-protective bag. This wear time may be extended past 30 days at the discretion of the unit commander. The suit may be worn for 24 hours in a contaminated area. Once the suit has been contaminated, the wearer must replace the suit by using the MOPP gear exchange procedure described in STP 21-1-SMCT, Soldier's Manual of Common Tasks, October 1990, Task # 031-503-1023, Exchange MOPP Gear. The discarded BDO must be incinerated or buried.

The BDO and DBDO are presently produced in both woodland and desert camouflage patterns. The suits have large butyl rubber patches sewn into the elbows and knees to prevent liquid chemical agents from penetrating the suit at these points.

The BDO and DBDO add approximately 11 pounds to the weight already carried by the soldier. In addition, the BDO prevents heat exchange with the environment and may add, depending on the wearer's level of exertion, 10EF to 15EF to his ambient temperature and heat burden. When wearing the BDO or DBDO at MOPP 1 or MOPP 2 and complete encapsulation is not required, certain modifications to the uniform are authorized:

- The trouser leg closures may be unzipped.
- The waist tabs may be loosened.
- The jacket may be unzipped.
- The sleeve Velcro closures may be opened.

This overall loosening of the BDO/DBDO will allow heat to escape as walking and other movements induce a bellows action of the suit against underlying clothing and skin. Because of the weight of the BDO/DBDO, field suspenders (8440-00-221-0852) should be used to allow support of the trousers and as much comfort as is possible.

Chemical Protective Gloves and Overboots

Gloves, 0.025-inch thickness

8415-01-144-1862 - X-Small
8415-01-033-3517 - Small
8415-01-033-3518 - Medium
8415-01-033-3519 - Large
8415-01-033-3520 - X-Large

Gloves, 0.014-inch thickness

8415-01-138-2497 - Small
8415-01-138-2498 - Medium

8415-01-138-2499 - Large
8415-01-138-2500 - X-Large

Gloves, Tactile 0.007-inch thickness

8415-01-138-2501 - Small
8415-01-138-2502 - Medium
8415-01-138-2503 - Large
8415-01-138-2504 - X-Large

Green Vinyl Overboots (GVO)

8430-01-048-6305 - Size 3
8430-01-048-6306 - Size 4
8430-01-049-0878 - Size 5
8430-01-049-0879 - Size 6
8430-01-049-0880 - Size 7
8430-01-049-0881 - Size 8
8430-01-049-0882 - Size 9
8430-01-049-0883 - Size 10
8430-01-049-0884 - Size 11
8430-01-049-0885 - Size 12
8430-01-049-0886 - Size 13

The chemical protective gloves are made from butyl rubber and are impermeable to chemical agents. The GVO is made from vinyl, which will protect the wearer against NBC agents and environmental effects. Both may also be decontaminated and reissued. Both the 0.025-inch thick and 0.014-inch thick gloves and GVO boots, when worn with the leather combat boot, can be used for 24 hours in a contaminated environment. After a complete visual inspection and decontamination with a 5% HTH solution, they may be worn again. The 0.007-inch thick **tactile** gloves must be inspected and decontaminated with the 5% HTH solution within 6 hours after being in a contaminated environment. Once decontaminated, the 0.007-inch thick **tactile** gloves may be re-used. In an uncontaminated environment, the gloves and boots can be used for 14 days, and if found to be serviceable after a thorough inspection, can be used for 14 days more. When working with petroleum products, care must be taken not to allow these products to contact the boots and gloves. Should petroleum products contaminate the boots and gloves, wipe off and air-dry the boots or gloves within two minutes. If this cannot happen within two minutes, new boots or gloves must be obtained immediately.

The green vinyl overboots are authorized for wear in a contaminated environment, but when the green vinyl is contaminated by a liquid agent, the agent will desorb as a vapor over a prolonged period of time. Decontamination of the rain boots while on chemically contaminated terrain would involve almost constant interruption of the mission and would in most cases be impractical. Therefore, the desorption of agent vapors from the GVO must be taken into account when conducting unmasking procedures or entrance procedures into a collective protection shelter.

The gloves and the boots pose safety hazards. The 0.025 inch thick and 0.014 inch thick gloves degrade tactile ability and in a cold environment will not provide adequate protection against cold injury. The 0.007-inch thick gloves have been produced to answer the need for **selected** personnel to have excellent tactile ability while wearing these gloves, but offer no protection from cold. These thin gloves must be issued along with the 0.025-inch thick gloves and only worn while performing those tasks requiring good tactile use of the hands and fingers.

For further information on these items, see FM 3-4, NBC Protection, 29 May 1992, Chapter 1. Individual Protective Equipment.

INDIVIDUAL DECONTAMINATION

The preceding section provided an overview of the primary items of chemical defense equipment which, when used correctly, will prevent contact with agent in typical battlefield concentrations. The problem of decontamination arises when some soldiers, because of bad training, bad discipline, or bad luck, become exposed to liquid agent despite the availability of protective masks and clothing.

This section addresses the two skin decontamination kits and the equipment decontamination kit currently in the inventory.

The kits are fairly simple in design and function, and instructions for their use are straightforward and easily committed to memory. Because of the potency of liquid nerve agents and the rapidly occurring tissue damage caused by vesicants, every soldier must be able to conduct an effective decontamination of all exposed skin automatically and without referring to the instructions printed on the kits.

The kits are as follows:

- Decontamination Kit, Skin: M291
- Decontamination Kit, Individual Equipment, M295
- Decontamination Kit, Skin: M258A1

Decontaminating Kit, Skin: M291

4230-01-276-1905

TM 3-4230-229-10

The introduction of this kit marks a new approach to skin decontamination. The M291 Kit consists of six identical packets, each containing a mixture of activated resins. This resin mixture both adsorbs liquid chemical agents present on the soldier's skin and neutralizes agents. The mixture consists of an adsorbent resin, a resin containing sulfonic acid, and a hydroxylamine-containing resin. After masking, the soldier opens any packet from the kit, removes the applicator pad, and applies an even coating of resin powder while scrubbing the entire skin area suspected to be contaminated. One applicator pad will decontaminate both hands and the face, if necessary. If the face must be decontaminated, then the neck (including the throat area) and the ears must also be decontaminated using a second applicator pad.

The black resin powder residue will provide a visual confirmation of the thoroughness of application and will not cause any skin irritation even after prolonged contact with skin. However, normal precautions must be observed so that the powder does not enter open wounds, the mouth, or the eyes. This kit will also be used for training; no training aid will be produced. The issue is 20 M291 Skin Decon Kits per box.

Decontamination Kit, Individual Equipment: M295 (DKIE)

4230-01-357-8456

TM 3-4230-235-10

The M295 DKIE allows for the decontamination of individual equipment through physical removal and absorption of chemical agent with no long-term, harmful side effects. The kit consists of a carrying pouch containing four individual decon packets, enough to do two complete individual equipment decontaminations. Each packet contains a mitt filled with the same decon powder used in the M291 skin decontamination kit. Two packets will decontaminate the protective gloves, M16A2 rifle, chemical protective helmet cover, protective mask hood, load carrying equipment (LCE) and accessories, mask carrying case, and protective boots.

The decon mitt will only remove surface liquid contamination. The equipment that has been decontaminated can still pose a vapor hazard, due to absorbed liquid chemical agent desorbing as a vapor.

The M295 DKIE will be issued to the squad at its lowest point of issue. The M295 DKIE is packaged in a "squad box" with 80 kits in each box. The squad members should be given at least one kit, and the packets for a complete decontamination can be carried in the cargo pocket of the BDO trouser.

As with the M291 SDK, the M295 DKIE will be used for both training and combat.

Decontamination Kit, Skin: M258A1

4230-01-101-3984

Training Aid, Skin Decontaminating: M58A1

6910-01-101-1768
6910-01-113-2434 - Refill Kit M58A1

TM 3-4230-216-10

The M258A1 skin decontamination kit is currently the standard item for the removal and neutralization of liquid chemical agents on the skin. This kit contains three No. 1 packets and three No. 2 packets. Packet No. 1 adsorbs and neutralizes the G-type nerve agents, whereas Packet No. 2 adsorbs and neutralizes the nerve agent VX and liquid mustard. The contents of the packets are as follows:

Packet No. 1	Packet No. 2
Hydroxyethane 72(+ or - 2)%	Chloramine B
Phenol 10 (+ or - 0.5)%	Hydroxyethane 45(+ or - 2)%
Sodium Hydroxide 5(+ or - 0.5)%	Zinc Chloride 5(+ or - 0.5)%
Ammonia 0.2 " 0.05%	Water
Water	

The soldier must remember that when using packet Number 1, one full minute of wiping the contaminated area is needed. The soldier must also remember that wiping with packet Number 2 must continue for two minutes. Speed and accuracy are critical in the proper use of this kit, and the soldier must have committed the decontamination procedure to memory. The decontamination solution is a skin-burn hazard in sensitive areas of the body and must be kept out of the eyes, mouth, and any open wounds. The kit must also be protected from freezing and prolonged exposure to temperatures greater than 110°F, and the glass ampoules in Packet No. 2 must be protected from premature breakage, which could render the kit useless. None of these disadvantages characterize the M291 Kit, which will soon replace the M258A1 Kit.

The M58A1 training aid was developed to avoid unnecessary exposure to the caustic components of the M258A1 Kit during training and is used in the same manner as the M258A1 skin decontamination kit. The training aid and the decontamination kit are distinguished by packaging color. The M258A1 Kit contains olive drab packets in an olive drab plastic case, whereas the M58A1 training aid contains blue packets in a black plastic case. The content of the M58A1 packets is 2-propanol and water.

For further information on these items see FM 3-4, page 124, and FM 3-5, NBC Decontamination, 17 November 1993, Chapter 2.

DETECTION AND ALARMS

This section will describe the equipment issued for detection and identification of chemical agent liquid and vapor in the environment. For both the individual soldier and the unit, these items of equipment are the primary means of identifying the presence and type of chemicals on the battlefield and of determining when a safe condition exists.

These equipment items are as follows:

- Paper, CM Agent Detector: M8
- Paper, CM Agent Detector: M9
- Chemical Agent Detector Kit: M256A1
- Chemical Agent Monitor
- Automatic Chemical Agent Alarm: M8A1
- Water Test Kit, Chemical Agents: M272

Paper, CM Agent Detector: M8

6665-00-050-8529

The use of M8 detector paper is the only way of identifying the type of chemical agent present in liquid form on the battlefield. Each soldier carries one booklet of M8 paper in the interior pocket of the protective mask carrier. A soldier encountering an unknown liquid suspected of being a chemical agent must don and check his mask and don the attached hood within 15 seconds, alert others in the vicinity, and then proceed to put on all of his chemical protective clothing. He then removes the booklet of M8 paper from his mask carrier, tears a half sheet from the booklet, and, if possible, affixes the sheet to a stick. Using the stick as a handle, the soldier then blots the paper onto the unknown liquid and waits for 30 seconds for a color change. The resulting color may then be compared to the colors on the inside of the front cover of the booklet to identify the type of liquid agent encountered.

- G: Nonpersistent Nerve: Yellow
- H: Blister: Red
- V: Persistent Nerve: Olive Green or Black

False positive can occur if liquid insecticides are on the surface being tested. Antifreeze and petroleum products will also cause false positive readings.

Paper, CM Agent Detector: M9

6665-01-049-8982

TM 3-4230-229-10

The M9 detector paper detects the presence of liquid chemical agent, but does not identify either the specific agent or the type of agent encountered. Each soldier carries one 30-feet long and 2-inch wide roll of M9 paper with adhesive backing to facilitate wrapping a strip of the paper around a sleeve and a trouser leg of the BDO. (Because the indicator dye in the paper is a potential carcinogen, gloves should be worn during application, and the paper should not contact the skin.) The paper is a dull, off-white or cream color in the absence of liquid agent but contains an indicator chemical that, when dissolved in liquid agent, turns a reddish color. When the soldier sees this color change, he must immediately mask, alert others, and if there is any possibility of skin exposure, proceed immediately with skin decontamination.

The M9 paper will detect nerve agent or blister agent droplets as small as 100 microns in diameter. False positive may be seen if the paper is exposed to antifreeze, liquid insecticide, or petroleum products. The soldier's attention to possible interfering substances on the battlefield can help in the later interpretation of a color change in the M9 paper in the absence of confirmation tests for agents. This does not relieve him of the obligation to mask and take other appropriate measures immediately after seeing a color change in the detector paper.

Chemical Agent Detector Kit: M256A1

6665-01-133-4964

TM 3-6665-307-10

Simulator, Detector Tickets, Chemical Agents: Training, M256A1

6665-01-112-1644

TM 3-6665-320-10

The M256A1 Chemical Agent Detection Kit is designed to detect and identify chemical agents present either as liquid or as vapor and consists of the following:

- a booklet of M8 paper (previously described) to detect agents in liquid form and

- 12 foil-wrapped detector tickets containing eel enzymes as reagents to detect very low concentrations of chemical vapors.

Instructions for the use of the detector tickets appear on the outside of each of the foil packets and in a separate instruction booklet in the kit. The following chart shows the agents detected by the M256A1 Kit.

Agent Detected	Symbol	Class
Hydrogen Cyanide	AC	"Blood" (cyanide)
Cyanogen Chloride	CK	"Blood" (cyanide)
Mustard	H	Blister
Nitrogen Mustard	HN	Blister
Distilled Mustard	HD	Blister
Phosgene Oxime	CX	Blister
Lewisite	L	Blister
Nerve Agents	V and G Series	Nerve

By following the directions on the foil packets or in the instruction booklet, a soldier can conduct a complete test with the liquid-sensitive M8 paper and the vapor-sensitive detector ticket in approximately 20 minutes. During the test, the ticket must be kept out of direct sunlight, which speeds evaporation of the reagents. Waving the detector ticket in the air also accelerates evaporation, so the ticket should be held stationary during all parts of the test.

The M256A1 trainer simulator was developed to provide realistic training while avoiding unnecessary exposure to potentially carcinogenic reagents in the

M256A1 detector kit. The M256A1 trainer contains 36 pre-engineered detector tickets and an instruction booklet. The pre-engineered detector tickets show color changes comparable to those seen when the M256A1 detector kit is used in clean or contaminated environments. Each training aid detector ticket has a specific code printed on the outside of the foil package. A list of codes is also printed on the inside of the training aid box under the lid, and instructions for the use of the simulator are also included. The codes are shown in the chart that follows.

MARK	*SIMULATED TEST FOR*
T-400	SAFE, "ALL CLEAR" - No NERVE, BLISTER, or BLOOD agents
T-401	DANGER - NERVE: G agents or VX
T-402	DANGER - BLISTER: HD (sulfur mustard)
T-403	DANGER - BLISTER: CX (phosgene oxime)
T-404	DANGER - BLOOD: AC (hydrogen cyanide) or CK (cyanogen chloride). (STRONG RXN indicates AC or CK in HIGH CONC)
T-404A	DANGER - BLOOD: AC (hydrogen cyanide) or CK (cyanogen chloride). (WEAK RXN indicates AC or CK in LOW CONC)

Chemical Agent Monitor (CAM)

6665-01-199-4153

TM 3-6665-331-12&P

The CAM, which is used to detect nerve and blister agents as vapors only, uses a 10-mCi nickel-63 (Ni^{63}) beta-particle radiation source to ionize airborne agent molecules that have been drawn into the unit by a pump. The resulting ion clusters vary in mass and charge and thus also travel at different rates in an applied electrical field. Comparison of the mobilities of the different ionic species to electronically stored standards allows an on-board microcomputer to determine the type of agent and its relative concentration. A liquid crystal display (LCD) presents these data as a series of concentration-dependent bars in a G mode for G agents and VX and in an H mode for blister agents.

The CAM detects agent vapor in that volume of air drawn by the pump into the sampling chamber of the instrument. It follows that the inlet port must not come into contact with a suspected area of evaporating agent on a surface but must nevertheless approach within a few inches of the site of suspected contamination. Because of the variation in agent concentration from one spot to another, depending upon wind velocity and other environmental factors, numerical displays of agent concentration in typical units would be impractical and unreliable. Accordingly, the display warns of a low vapor hazard (1 to 3 bars visible), a high vapor hazard (4 to 6 bars visible), or a very high vapor hazard (7 to 8 bars visible).

Chemical Agent Alarm: M8A1

6665-01-105-5623

TM 3-6665-312-12&P

The M8A1 Automatic Chemical Agent Alarm (ACAA) is the only remote continuous air sampling alarm in the U.S. Army at present. This alarm will sample the air for the presence of NERVE agent vapors (GA, GB, GD, and VX) only. The M8A1 alarm uses 0.01 millicurie of americium-241 (Am^{241}), a source of alpha particles to ionize airborne agent molecules drawn into the sampling chamber by a pump module. A detector cell analyzes the resulting ion clusters and compares their masses and charges with electronically stored standards to detect the presence of nerve agent vapors. The operator may specify whether the alarm itself is audible, visual, or both.

The system consists of the M43A1 detector, as many as five M42 alarm units, and various power supplies. The detector cell and alarm units are most commonly found in a fixed-site configuration. Normally the M43A1 detectors are placed facing into the wind no more than 150 meters outside the unit perimeter, with no more than 300 meters between detectors, and when possible, no more than 400 meters between the detector cells and the alarm units. WD-1/TT 6145-00-226-8812 telephone cable connects the detector cells and the alarm units. The alarm units are placed throughout the facility. A typical Mobile Army Surgical Hospital (MASH) has three M8A1 ACAAs, and a Combat Support Hospital (CSH) has seven M8A1 ACAAs.

Water Testing Kit, Chemical Agents: M272

6665-01-134-0885

TM 3-6665-319-10

The M272 water test kit was designed and fielded to answer the need for a test to detect water contamination by nerve agent, blister agent, cyanide ("blood" agent), or Lewisite. The kit will operate between 32EF and 125EF. An enclosed instruction card enables a soldier to conduct all the tests required to identify the threat agents. The kit will detect the chemical agents at the concentrations indicated in the chart that follows.

Chemical Agent	*Symbol(s)*	*Concentration (mg/l)-**
Cyanide	AC	20.0 as CN^-
Mustard	HD	2.0 --
Lewisite	L	2.0 as As^{+++}
Nerve	G/V	0.02 --

*Concentration reliably detected by kit tests.

Water containing agents in lesser concentrations is permissible for short-term use (up to 7 days) in both cold and warm regions as long as the daily consumption per person does not exceed 5 quarts. Each kit contains enough reagents for tests on 25 separate water samples. The operator can easily conduct the full range of tests in 20 minutes when the temperature is between 50EF and 105EF; at lower temperatures, the water samples and the nerve agent ticket should both be warmed for 10 minutes before beginning testing. Water that is too hot may cause foaming in the detector tubes for Lewisite, mustard, and cyanide; therefore, water at temperatures between 105EF and 125EF should be cooled for at least 5 minutes to reduce its temperature to 105E or cooler.

PATIENT PROTECTIVE EQUIPMENT

In this section, the following three items that have been fielded will be discussed:

- Patient Protective Wrap
- Decontaminable Litter
- Resuscitation Device Individual Chemical (RDIC)

Patient Protective Wrap

8456-01-079-9875

Army Medical Department (AMEDD) doctrine calls for the treatment as far forward as possible of casualties from the integrated battlefield. Because treatment often mandates removal of the BDO and precludes donning replacement BDOs, a patient protective wrap has been developed. This wrap is sturdy and lightweight, weighing approximately 2.7 kg, and it protects the patient from all known chemical agents for up to six continuous hours. It is not designed for use by more than one patient and must be discarded after use.

One continuous zipper around the outer edge of the top sheet provides easy patient insertion into the wrap, and observation of the patient is possible through an impermeable transparent window at the head of the wrap. Below the window, a small transparent pocket is large enough to hold a field medical card or other medical record, and two protected sleeves next to the window permit the passage of IV tubing.

The wrap is designed for use on a litter but can itself become a field-expedient litter if necessary. Along the sides of the wrap are sleeves through which poles can be inserted. These sleeves have handholds for manual carries when poles are not available. It is recommended that the patient wear the mask while in the wrap, but this is not a requirement; however, before the casualty is put into the wrap, a cardboard insert must first be placed into the wrap to hold the window material away from the patient's face.

Although the protective wrap is permeable to both oxygen and carbon dioxide, the rate at which carbon dioxide is produced by a typical patient exceeds by a small amount the rate at which this gas passes through the wrap. Therefore, the patient should not be left in the wrap for longer than the recommended maximum of six hours.

Decontaminable Litter

6530-01-290-9964

Contaminated casualties arriving at a medical treatment location will in most cases require decontamination prior to definitive treatment. This decontamination process will require the use of the limited supplies of equipment organic to the treatment unit. Ideally, equipment in limited supply should be capable of complete decontamination using field-available methods. However, in tests conducted by the U.S. Army Soldier and Biological Chemical Command, canvas litters exposed to liquid blister agents and then decontaminated still desorbed vapors for 72 hours after all surface contaminants were removed.

The decontaminable litter was thus developed to replace the canvas litters currently in use. The new litter is made from a monofilament polypropylene that has high tensile strength and low elasticity. The fabric does not absorb liquid chemical agents and is not degraded by decontaminating solutions. The fabric is flame retardant, highly rip resistant, and treated to withstand exposure to weather and sunlight. The fabric has a honeycomb weave which results in a rough, non-slip surface, and liquids easily pass through the 40% of the surface area that is open. The carrying handles retract into the metal pole frame for a closed total length of 83.5 inches (212.1 cm) to allow for loading the litter onto the UH-60 helicopter. The handles have TWO open positions, 90.0 inches

(228.1 cm) and 91.6 inches (232.7 cm). The first position is a NATO standard, and the second position was provided to allow increased gripping comfort by litter bearers. The aluminum poles have been designed to provide direct gripping surfaces for litter stanchions. All metal parts have been painted with Chemical Agent Resistant Coating (CARC) paint.

Resuscitation Device, Individual Chemical

6665-01-338-6602

The Resuscitation Device, Individual Chemical (RDIC) is a ventilatory system consisting of a compressible butyl rubber bag, a NATO standard C2 canister filter, a nonrebreathing valve, a cricothyroid cannula adapter. and a flexible hose connected to an oropharyngeal mask. The mask is removable from the distal end of the flexible hose for connection of the hose to the cannula adapter. The butyl rubber bag resists the penetration of liquid chemical agent that may be on the chemical protective gloves of operator and is easily decontaminated. The elasticity of the outer cover limits airway pressure to a maximal value of 70 cm H_2O (70 mbar). The device will deliver up to 600 ml of filtered air per cycle at a rate of 30 cycles per minute.

The RDIC will be fielded one per air ambulance, one per ground ambulance, and one per Chemical Agent Treatment, MES.

APPENDIX A

PATIENT DECONTAMINATION

OVERVIEW

Patient decontamination is personnel, time, and equipment intensive. Nevertheless, with a little ingenuity and attention to just a few basic principles, an effective litter decontamination procedure can be accomplished with minimal cost. The first part of this appendix briefly discusses considerations in establishing a decontamination site, followed by step-by-step procedures.

The decontamination site is part of the medical treatment facility, and the same considerations for establishing the treatment facility apply to the decontamination area. The decontamination area is located about 50 yards downwind from the treatment area (i.e., wind blowing from the clean treatment area to the dirty decontamination area).

KEY PRINCIPLES

- Wind direction
- Security of the decontamination site
- Area control of the decontamination site
- Litter patient decontamination
- Ambulatory patient decontamination

The important considerations of personnel and equipment requirements are discussed in other publications.

Wind Direction

Wind direction is important because a vapor hazard may be present downwind from a liquid contaminated area (i.e., patient arrival/triage area). Patient decontamination is always performed upwind, or at least not downwind, from the patient arrival area.

The decontamination site will initially be set up to take advantage of the prevailing wind; however, setup should be adaptable to allow for quick rearrangement when the wind comes from another direction.

If the wind changes direction by more than 45°, the decontamination site will need to be adjusted accordingly. A wait of 15 to 20 minutes to determine if the change is permanent should precede the move. When the site is moved, it must be moved at least 75 meters upwind from any contaminated area. Personnel working in the old "clean" area when the wind shifts must ensure that all casualties remain masked. This scenario points out that the ideal decontamination setup should include 2 separate decontamination sites approximately 75 meters apart, when possible.

Security of Decontamination Site

When choosing a decontamination site, the same security considerations must be given as for any other site chosen for medical operations. The decontamination site is at the same potential risk from attack as is the actual medical treatment facility.

Area Control of Decontamination Site

An entry control point (ECP) can be established to control movement of clean and contaminated vehicles to the Medical Treatment Facility (MTF) or the Decontamination Site. The ECP should be located at a distance far enough from the MTF to keep vapor hazard from contaminated vehicles to the minimum.

Traffic control at the decontamination site involves routing a clearly marked, one-way course from the ECP to the decontamination site.

Control of personnel movement is necessary to ensure that contaminated walking personnel do not accidentally contaminate clean areas. The hot line must be secured. Concertina wire works well to keep personnel in the desired areas, and a clearly marked, one-way route helps to ensure that correct entry and exit points are used.

LITTER PATIENT DECONTAMINATION

Personnel

Two people are required per litter patient. These two augmentees will link up with one litter patient in the triage area and work with that same litter patient until hand-off at the "hot line." These two people conduct both clothing removal and any required skin decontamination. To assist these two augmentees, two other augmentees will be needed, one to assist the first two augmentees in picking up the patient from the clothing removal litter, and the second to remove the contaminated clothing and litter and replace it with a clean litter. These four augmentees will conduct all patient decontamination and movement of the patient while in MOPP level IV and the Toxicological Agent Protective (TAP) apron.

Personnel working in the patient decontamination area will be at MOPP level IV plus the Toxicological Agent Protective (TAP) apron. At least two people from this area will move to the triage area and carry the patient from this area to the first decontamination station.

Hypochlorite Solutions

Two different concentrations of chlorine solution are used in the patient decontamination procedure. A 0.5% chlorine solution is used for all patient washing procedures and for the mask decontamination. The 5% chlorine solution is used to decontaminate the scissors, the TAP aprons, and the gloves on personnel working in the patient decontamination area and the casualty's hood. The chlorine solutions are placed in buckets for use in this area. The buckets should be distinctly marked because it is very difficult to tell the difference between the 5% and 0.5% chlorine solutions. These solutions may be made using the 6-ounce Calcium Hypochlorite (HTH) containers that come with the Chemical Agent Decon Set. The 0.5% solution can be made adding one 6-ounce container of calcium hypochlorite to 5 gallons of water. Adding eight 6-ounce containers of calcium hypochlorite to 5 gallons of water can make the 5% CL solution. These solutions evaporate quickly at high temperatures, so if they are made in advance, they should be stored in closed containers.

Procedure

1. Decontaminate the mask and hood. Sponge down front, sides, and top of hood with 5.0% calcium hypochlorite solution, or wipe off with the M258A1 or the M291 Decon Kit.

2. Remove hood.

a. Dip scissors in 5% HTH solution.
b. Cut off hood.
(1) Release or cut hood shoulder straps.
(2) Cut/untie neck cord.
(3) Cut/remove zipper cord.
(4) Cut/remove drawstring under the voicemitter.
(5) Unzip the hood zipper.
(6) Cut the cord away from the mask.
(7) Cut the zipper below the voicemitter.
(8) Proceed cutting upward, close to the inlet valve covers and eye lens outserts.
(9) Cut upward to top of eye lens outsert.
(10) Cut across forehead to the outer edge of the next eye lens outsert.
(11) Cut downward toward patient's shoulder staying close to the eye lens outsert inlet valve cover.

(12) Cut across the lower part of the voicemitter to the zipper.

(13) Dip scissors in HTH solution.

(14) Cut from center of forehead over the top of the head.

(15) Fold left and right sides of the hood to the side of the patient's head, laying sides on the litter.

c. The Quick Doff Hood is loosened and removed.

3. Decontaminate protective mask/face.

a. Use M258A1, M291, or 0.5% hypochlorite solution.

b. Cover both inlet valve covers with gauze or hands.

c. Wipe external parts of mask.

d. Uncover inlet valve covers.

e. Wipe exposed areas of patient's face.

(1) Chin

(2) Neck

(3) Back of ears

4. Remove Field Medical Card (FMC).

a. Cut the FMC tie wire.
b. Allow the FMC to fall into a plastic bag.
c. Seal plastic bag and wash with 0.5% hypochlorite solution.
d. Place plastic bag under back of mask head straps.

5. Remove all gross contamination from the patient's overgarment.

a. Wipe all evident contamination spots with M258A1 Decon Kit, M291, or 5% hypochlorite solution.
b. Wipe external parts of mask with M258A1 Decon Kit or M291.
c. Use wipe 1, then wipe 2, to clean exterior of mask; use wipe 2, then wipe 1 to clean interior.

6. Cut and remove overgarment. Cut clothing around tourniquets, bandages, and splints. Two people will be cutting clothing at the same time. Dip scissors in 5% hypochlorite solution before doing each complete cut to avoid contaminating inner clothing.

a. Cut overgarment jacket.
(1) Unzip protective overgarment.
(2) Cut from wrist area of sleeves, up to armpits, and then to neck area.

(3) Roll chest sections to respective sides with inner surface outward.

(4) Tuck clothing between arm and chest.

(5) Repeat procedure for other side of jacket.

b. Cut overgarment trousers.

(1) Cut from cuff along inseam to waist on left leg.

(2) On right overgarment leg, cut from cuff to just below zipper and then go sideways into the first cut.

(3) Allow trouser halves to drop to litter with contamination away from patient.

(4) Tuck trouser halves to sides of body and roll the camouflage sides under between the legs.

7. Remove outer gloves. This procedure can be done with one aidman on each side of the patient working simultaneously. Do not remove inner gloves.

a. Lift the patient's arms by grasping his gloves.

b. Fold the glove away from the patient over the sides of the litter.

c. Grasp the fingers of the glove.

d. Roll the cuff over the finger, turning the glove inside out.

e. Carefully lower the arm(s) across the chest when the glove(s) is removed. (Do not allow the arms to contact the exterior (camouflage side) of the overgarment.)

f. Dispose of contaminated gloves.
   (1) Place in plastic bag.
   (2) Deposit in contaminated dump.

g. Dip your own gloves in HTH solution.

8. Remove overboots.

a. Cut laces.
b. Fold lacing eyelets flat outward.
c. Hold heels with one hand.
d. Pull overboots downwards over the heels with other hand.
e. Pull towards you until removed.
f. Place overboots in contaminated disposal bag.

9. Remove personal articles from pockets.

a. Place in plastic bags.
b. Seal bags.
c. Place in contaminated holding area.

10. Remove combat boots without touching body surfaces.

a. Cut boot laces along the tongue.
b. Pull boots downward and toward you until removed.
c. Place boots in contaminated dump.

11. Remove inner clothing.

a. Unbuckle belt.

b. Cut battle dress uniform (BDU) pants following same procedures as for overgarment trousers.

c. Cut fatigue jacket following the same procedures as for overgarment jacket.

12. Remove undergarments following same procedure as for fatigues. If patient is wearing a brassiere, it is cut between cups. Both shoulder straps are cut where they attach to the cups and laid back off the shoulders.

13. __Clothing removal to skin decontamination__. Transfer the patient to a decontamination litter. After the patient's clothing has been cut away, he is transferred to a decontamination litter or a canvas litter with a plastic sheeting cover. Three decontamination team members decontaminate their gloves and apron with the 5% hypochlorite solution. One member places his hands under the small of the patient's legs and thigh, a second member places his arms under the patient's back and buttocks, and the third member places his arms under the patient's shoulders and supports the head and neck. They carefully lift the patient using their knees, not their backs, to minimize back strain. While the patient is elevated, another decontamination team member removes the litter from the litter stands and another member replaces it with a decontamination (clean)

litter. The patient is carefully lowered onto the clean litter. Two decontamination members carry the litter to the skin decontamination station. The contaminated clothing and overgarment are placed in bags and moved to the decontaminated waste dump. The dirty litter is rinsed with the 5% decontamination solution and placed in a litter storage area. Decontaminated litters are returned by ambulance to the maneuver units.

14. **Skin decontamination**. The areas of potential contamination should be spot decontaminated using the M258A1 kit, the M291 kit, or 0.5% hypochlorite solution. These areas include the neck, wrists, lower face, and skin under tears or holes in the protective ensemble. After the patient is decontaminated, his dressings and tourniquet are changed. Superficial (not body cavities, eyes, or nervous tissue) wounds are flushed with the 0.5% CL solution and new dressings are applied as needed. Cover massive wounds with plastic or plastic bags. New tourniquets are placed 0.5 to 1 inch proximal to the original tourniquet, and then the old tourniquets are removed. Splints are not removed but saturated to the skin with 0.5% CL solution. If the splint cannot be saturated (air splint or canvas splint), it must be removed sufficiently so that everything below the splint can be saturated with the 0.5% CL solution. The patient, his wounds, and the decontaminable stretcher have now been completely decontaminated.

15. <u>**Final monitoring and movement to treatment area**</u>. The patient is monitored for contamination using the Chemical Agent Monitor (CAM), M8 paper, or M9 paper. The contents of the M258A1 kit (pad 1 and pad 2 when used separately or together) and hypochlorite solution on the skin do not affect the CAM. However, pad 1 of the M258A1 kit causes M8 paper to turn dark green (V agent), pad 2 causes no color change, and the pads used together cause M8 paper to turn yellow (G agent). Each pad causes the M9 paper to react (turn red). Once the casualty is confirmed clean of chemical agent, he is transferred via a shuffle pit over the hot line. The shuffle pit is composed of two parts Super Tropical Bleach (STB) and three parts earth or sand. The shuffle pit should be deep enough to cover the bottom of the protective overboots. The buddy system wash of the TAP apron and gloves in 5.0% hypochlorite solution precedes the transfer of the patient to a new, clean canvas litter if the decontaminable stretchers are in limited supply. A three-person patient lift is again used as the litter is switched. If the litter as well as the patient was checked, both patient and the same litter can be placed over the hot line.

AMBULATORY PATIENT DECON

Casualties who are decontaminated in an ambulatory area are those who (1) require treatment that can be supplied in the emergency treatment area, or (2) require resupply of their protective overgarment in the clean area before return to duty. Those who require clothing removal use the litter decontamination procedure, as removal of clothing is not done in this area.

Personnel

Personnel from the decontamination station might assist the casualty, or the casualties might assist each other during this process under close supervision.

Procedure

Decontamination of ambulatory patients follows the same principles as for litter patients. The major difference is the sequence of clothing removal, listed below, to lessen the chance of the patient contaminating himself and others.

The first five steps are the same as in litter patient decontamination and are not described in detail.

1. Remove load-bearing equipment.

2. Decontaminate mask and hood and remove hood.

3. Decontaminate skin around mask.

4. Remove Field Medical Card and put it into a plastic bag.

5. Remove gross contamination from the outergarment; remove and bag personal effects from overgarment.

6. Overgarment Jacket Removal

a. Instruct patient to:
   (1) Clench his fist.
   (2) Stand with arms held straight down.
   (3) Extend arms backward at about a 30-degree angle.
   (4) Place feet shoulder width apart.

b. Stand in front of patient.
   (1) Untie drawstring.
   (2) Unsnap jacket front flap.
   (3) Unzip jacket front.

c. Move to the rear of the patient.
   (1) Grasp jacket collar at sides of the neck.
   (2) Peel jacket off shoulders at a 30-degree angle down and away from the patient.
   (3) Smoothly pull the inside of sleeves over the patient's wrists and hands.

d. Cut to aid removal if necessary.

7. Removal of Butyl Rubber Gloves

a. Patient's arms are still extended backward at a 30-degree angle.

(1) Dip your gloved hands in 5% hypochlorite solution.

(2) Use thumbs and forefingers of both hands.

(a) Grasp the heel of patient's glove at top and bottom of forearm.

(b) Peel gloves off with a smooth downward motion. This procedure can easily be done with one person or with one person on each side of the patient working simultaneously.

(c) Place gloves in contaminated disposal bag.

b. Tell the patient to reposition his arms, but not to touch his trousers.

8. Remove patient's overboots.

a. Cut overboot laces with scissors dipped in 5% hypochlorite solution.

b. Fold lacing eyelets flat on ground.

c. Step on the toe and heel eyelet to hold eyelets on the ground.

d. Instruct patient to step out of the overboot onto clean area. If in good condition, the overboot can be decontaminated and reissued.

9. Remove overgarment trousers.

a. Unfasten or cut all ties, buttons, or zippers.
b. Grasp trousers at waist.
c. Peel trousers down over the patient's boots.
d. Cut trousers to aid removal if necessary.
(1) Cut around all bandages and tourniquets.
(2) Cut from inside pant leg ankle to groin.
(3) Cut up both sides of the zipper to the waist.
(4) Allow the narrow strip with zipper to drop between the legs.
(5) Peel or allow trouser halves to drop to the ground.
e. Tell patient to step out of trouser legs one at a time.
f. Place trousers into contaminated disposal bag.

10. Remove glove inner liners. Patient should remove the liners since this will reduce the possibility of spreading contamination. Tell patient to remove white glove liners.

a. Grasp heel of glove without touching exposed skin.
b. Peel liner downward and off.
c. Drop in contaminated disposal.

d. Remove the remaining liner in the same manner.

e. Place liners in contaminated disposal bag.

11. Final monitoring and decontamination.

a. Monitor/test with M8 Detection Paper or CAM.

b. Check all areas of patient's clothing.

c. Give particular attention to:

(1) Discolored areas
(2) Damp spots
(3) Tears in clothing
(4) Neck
(5) Wrist
(6) Around dressings

d. Decontaminate all contamination on clothing or skin by cutting away areas of clothing or using 5% hypochlorite solution, the M291, or the M258A1 for clothing or 0.5% hypochlorite solution and the M291, or the M258A1 for skin.

12. The medical corpsman should remove bandages and tourniquets and decontaminate splints using the procedures described in the decontamination of a litter patient during overgarment removal.

13. The patient is decontaminated and ready to be moved inside the hot line. Instruct patient to shuffle

his feet to dust his boots thoroughly as he walks through the shuffle pit.

In the clean treatment area the patient can now be retriaged, treated, evacuated, etc. In a hot climate the patient will probably be significantly dehydrated, and the rehydration process should start.

Comments

The clean area is the resupply point for the patient decontamination site. Water is needed for rehydration of persons working in the decontamination area. The resupply section should have an adequate stock of canteens with the chemical cap.

A location is needed in each decontamination area (75 meters from the working decontamination site) to allow workers, after they have decontaminated their TAP aprons, to remove their masks and rehydrate. There are generally not enough battle dress overgarments (BDOs) available to allow workers to remove them during the rest cycle and don new gear before going back to work. If these clean/shaded rest areas are not provided, the workers must remain in MOPP IV even during rest periods, and water must be drunk through the mask via the drinking port. If all water consumption is by mask, there must be a canteen refill area adjacent to the vapor/clean line in which empty canteens can be decontaminated and placed for refill and clean full canteens are present for rehydration.

(The above procedures were adapted from FM 8-10-4 and FM 8-10-7.)

APPENDIX B

CASUALTY RECEIVING AREA

The diagram shows a set-up for casualty reception in a contaminated environment. The chapter on casualty management describes the stations.

The actual set-up of this area may vary depending on the assets and circumstances.

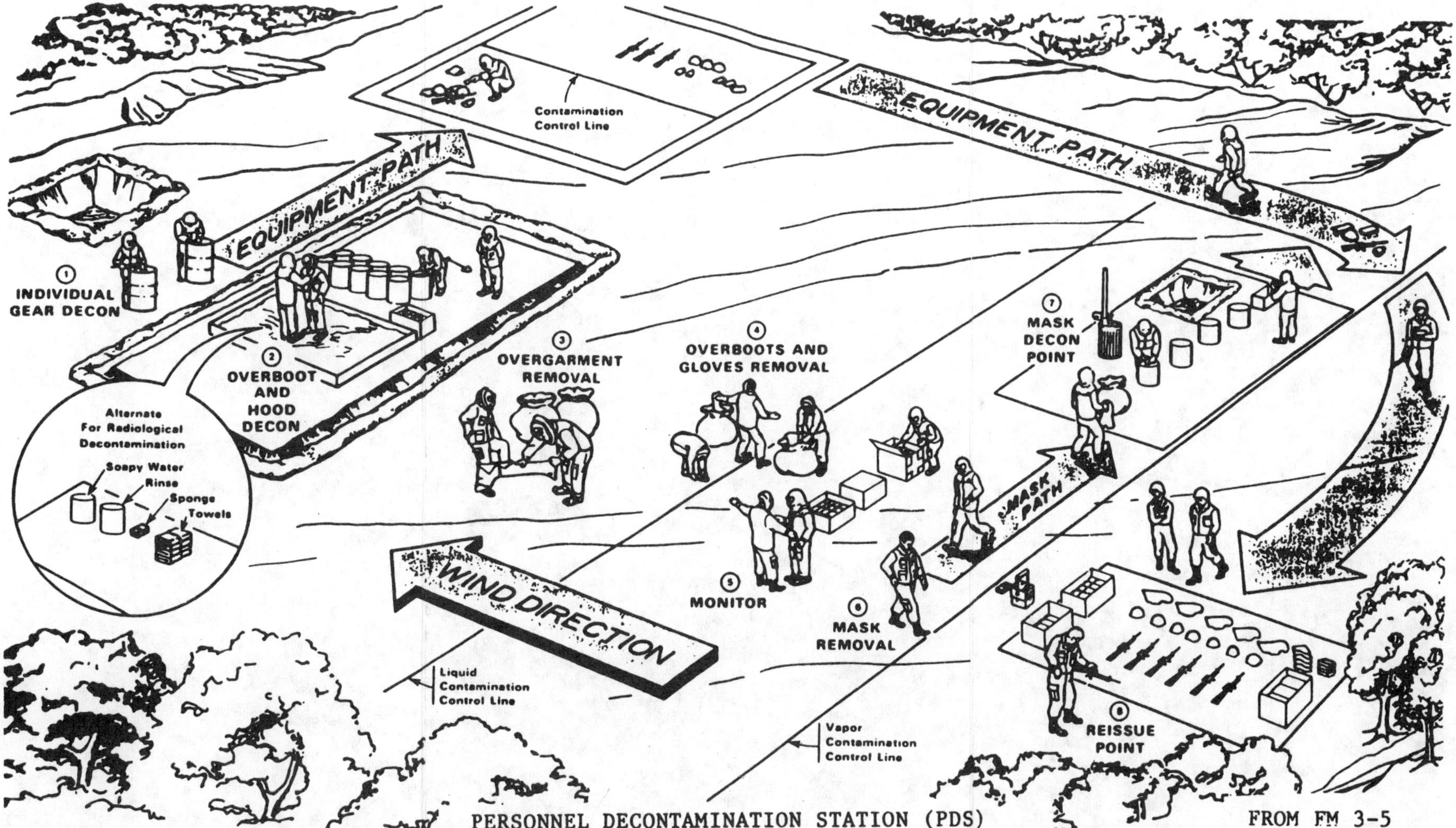

PERSONNEL DECONTAMINATION STATION (PDS)

FROM FM 3-5

APPENDIX C

PERSONNEL DECONTAMINATION STATION

The following foldout is a diagram of the Personnel Decontamination Station. This is a decontamination procedure for noncasualty personnel. It is not a medical specific procedure, but a procedure that all units in the military, including medical units, employ.

Using this procedure, contaminated, noncasualty personnel can move from the contaminated (dirty) area across the hot line to the non-contaminated (clean) area. In a medical unit, this procedure would be followed by those working in the dirty area (such as the triage officer, the decontamination team) moving to the clean area.

A related procedure (not shown) is the MOPP exchange station. In this station, personnel who have been wearing contaminated MOPP gear longer than the recommended time can exchange their dirty protective garments for clean garments.

(Taken from FM 3-5.)

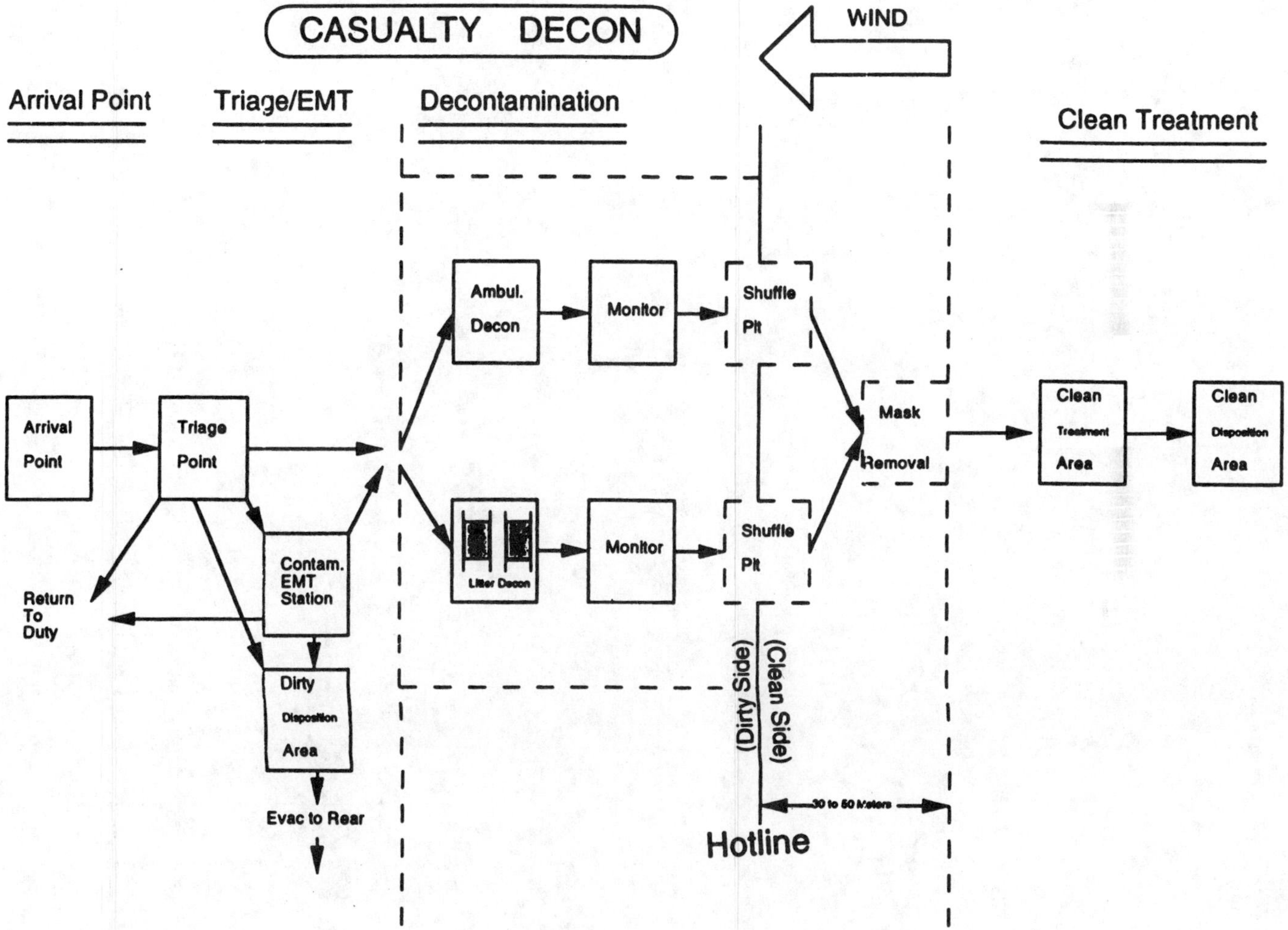

CASUALTY DECON
WIND
Arrival Point
Triage/EMT
Decontamination
Clean Treatment
Arrival Point
Triage Point
Return To Duty
Contam. EMT Station
Dirty Disposition Area
Evac to Rear
Ambul. Decon
Litter Decon
Monitor
Monitor
Shuffle Pit
Shuffle Pit
Mask Removal
(Dirty Side)
(Clean Side)
30 to 50 Meters
Hotline
Clean Treatment Area
Clean Disposition Area

APPENDIX D

TOXICITY DATA

The following tables provide estimated human toxicity data on the agents discussed in this Handbook.

Agent	Effect	Ct_{50} (mg-min/m^3)	Liquid on skin
GA	Miosis	~2-3	
	Death	200-400	
GB	Miosis	~3	
	Death	100-200	
GD	Miosis	~2-3	
	Death	50-70	
VX	Death	10-50	
HD	Eye	12-200	

Agent	Effect	Ct_{50} (mg-min/m^3)	Liquid on skin
HD	Pulmonary	100-200	
	Erythema	200-1000	10 μg
	Death	1500 inhalation 10,000 skin	100 mg/kg
L	Erythema	>1500	10-15 μg
	Death	~1500 inhalation	40-50 mg/kg
CX	Eye	200?	
	Erythema	2500?	
	Death	3200?	
CG	Pulmonary effects	>1600	
	Death	3200	
AC	Death	2500-5000	
CK	Death	11,000	

Agent	Effect	Ct_{50} (mg-min/m^3)
CN	Irritation	10-20
	Death	14,000
CS	Irritation	5-10
	Death	>50,000

APPENDIX E

PHYSICOCHEMICAL DATA

The following tables provide physicochemical data on the agents discussed in this Handbook.

	GA *Tabun*	GB *Sarin*	GD *Soman*	GF	VX
Molecular Weight	162	140	182	180	267
Vapor Density	5.63	4.86	6.33	6.2	9.2
Liquid Density	1.07@ 25°C	1.09@ 25°C	1.02@ 25°C	1.17@ 20°C	1.01@ 20°C
Freezing/ Melting Point (°C)	-5	-56	-42	-30	<-51
Boiling Point (°C)	240	158	198	239	298
Vapor Pressure	0.037	2.9	0.4	0.04	0.007
Volatility	610	22,000	3,900	438	10.5

	HD *(Distilled Mustard)*	**L** *(Lewisite)*	**CX** *(Phosgene Oxime)*
Molecular Weight	159	207	114
Vapor Density	5.4	7.1	3/9
Liquid Density	1.27@25°C	1.89@20°C	--
Freezing/Melting Point (°C)	14	-18	35-40
Boiling Point (°C)	217	190	53-54
Vapor Pressure	0.07@20°C	0.39@20°C	11.2@25°C
Volatility	610@20°C	4480@20°C	1800@20°C

	AC *(Hydrogen Cyanide)*	CK *(Cyanogen Choride)*	CG *(Phosgene Oxime)*
Molecular Weight	27	61	99
Vapor Density	0.99	2.1	3.4
Liquid Density	0.69	1.18	1.37
Freezing/Melting Point (°C)	-13.3	-6.9	-128
Boiling Point (°C)	25.7	12.8	7.6
Vapor Pressure	742@25°C	1000@25°C	1.17@20°C
Volatility	1,080,000@ 25°C	2,600,000@ 12.8°C	4,300,000 @7.6°C

	CN *(Mace)*	CS
Molecular Weight	155	189
Vapor Density	5.3	--
Liquid Density	1.32 (solid) @20°C	1.04@20°C
Freezing/Melting Point (°C)	54	˜94
Boiling Point (°C)	249	˜310 (with decomposition)
Vapor Pressure	0.0041@20°C	0.00034@20°C
Volatility	34.3@20°C	0.71@25°C

APPENDIX F

MEDICAL EQUIPMENT SET CHEMICAL AGENT PATIENT TREATMENT

NOMENCLATURE/NSN	AMOUNT
Atropine, Inj. 0.70L/6505-00-926-9083	500 ea
Pralidoxime Chloride/6505-01-125-3248	100 ea
Boric Acid 5%/6505-01-153-3012	36 tu
Sodium Nitrite/6505-01-206-6009	12 pg
Sodium Thiosulfate/6505-01-206-6010	12 pg
Diazepam/6505-01-274-0951	3 pg
Atropine Sulfate/6505-01-332-1281	1 pg
Infusion Set Size: 2/6515-00-089-2791	60 ea
Airway Pharyn LGE/6515-00-300-2900	6 ea
Airway Pharyn SM/6515-00-300-2910	6 ea

NOMENCLATURE/NSN	AMOUNT
Syringe Hypo 10 ml/6515-00-754-0412	.6 pg
Needle Hypo 18 ga/6515-00-754-2834	1.2 bx
Suction Apparatus/6515-01-076-3577	4 ea
Resuscitator Hand/6515-01-338-6602	4 ea
Syringe Hypo 50 ml/6515-01-280-2320	1 pg
Chest No. 4/6545-00-914-3490	3 ea
Gloves'Chem/8415-01-138-2502	2 pr
Gloves Chem/8415-01-138-2503	2 pr
Bag Chem Cas/8465-01-079-9875	12 ea

MEDICAL EQUIPMENT SET

CHEMICAL AGENT PATIENT DECONTAMINATION

NOMENCLATURE/NSN	AMOUNT
M291 SDK/4230-01-276-1905	2 bx
Bandage Scissors/6515-00-935-7138	6 ea
Syringe Hypo/6515-01-280-2320	.6 pg
Litter Support/6530-00-660-0034	4 pr
Chest No. 4/6545-00-914-3490	1 ea
Chest No. 6/6545-00-914-3510	1 ea
M9 Chem Agt Paper/6665-01-049-8982	1 ro
Calcium Hypo/6810-00-255-0471	48 bo
12 qt Pail/7240-00-773-0975	10 ea
Sponge Cellulose/7920-00-884-1115	6 ea
Bag Plastic/8105-00-191-3902	2 ro

NOMENCLATURE/NSN	AMOUNT
Plastic Sheet/8135-00-618-1783	2 ro
Work Gloves MED/8415-00-268-8353	25 pr
Work Gloves SM/8415-00-258-8354	25 pr
Black Pencils/7510-00-240-1526	2 dz
TAP Apron SM/8415-00-281-7813	2 ea
TAP Apron MED/8415-00-281-7814	4 ea
TAP Apron LRG/8415-00-281-7815	2 ea
Chem Prot Glove/8415-01-033-3517	2 ea
Chem Prot Glove/8415-01-033-3518	4 ea
Chem Prot Glove/8415-01-033-3519	2 ea
Decon Litter/6530-01-290-9964	4 ea

APPENDIX G

The following table is intended to serve as a reminder of the agents, their effects, first-aid measures, detection, and skin decontamination.

It is in no way complete, nor is it intended to be complete. Consult the appropriate chapter for further details.

Type of Agent	Effects	Onset	First-aid	Skin Decon	Detection
Pulmonary: CG (PFIB), HC	Dyspnea, coughing	Hours	None	None usually needed	None
Cyanide: AC, CK	Loss of consciousness, convulsions, apnea	Seconds	None (nitrite and thiosulfate)	None usually needed	M256A1
Vesicants: H, HD, L	Erythema, blisters; irritation of eyes; cough, dyspnea	Hours (immediate pain after L)	None	M291, M258A1, bleach, water	M256A1, M8 and M9 papers, CAM

Type of Agent	Effects	Onset	First-aid	Skin Decon	Detection
Nerve: GA, GB, GD, GF, VX	Vapor: miosis, rhinorrhea, dyspnea Liquid: sweating, vomiting Both: convulsions, apnea	Seconds Minutes to hours	MARK I (1 to 3), diazepam	M291, M258A1, bleach, water	M8A1 alarm, M256A1, M8 and M9 papers, CAM
Incapacitating: BZ, Agent 15	Mydriasis, dry mouth and skin; confusion, visual hallucinations	Hours	None	Water, soap and water	None
Riot-control: CS, CN	Burning, stinging of eyes, nose, airways, skin	Seconds	None	Water	None

APPENDIX H

GLOSSARY OF TERMS

ACAA: Automatic Chemical Agent Alarm

AMEDD: Army Medical Department

BDO: Battle Dress Overgarment

BDU: Battle Dress Uniform

CAM: Chemical Agent Monitor

CANA: Convulsive Antidote, Nerve Agent

CARC: Chemical Agent Resistant Coating

C/B: Chemical/Biological

CDC: Chemical Decontamination Center

CBPS: Chemical and Biological Protective Shelter

CPS: Chemical Protective Shelter

DAAMS: Depot Area Air Monitoring System

DBDO: Desert Battle Dress Overgarment

DTD: Detailed Troop Decontamination

ECP: Entry Control Point

FMC: Field Medical Card

GREGG: Graves Registration

HTH: High Test Hypochlorite

KPH: Kilometer Per Hour

ICAD: Individual Chemical Agent Monitor

LBE: Load Bearing Equipment

LCL: Liquid Control Line

MES: Medical Equipment Set

MOPP: Mission Oriented Protective Posture

MTF: Medical Treatment Facility

MTO&E: Modified Table of Organization and Equipment

NAAK: Nerve Agent Antidote Kit

NATO: North Atlantic Treaty Organization

NBC: Nuclear/Biological/Chemical

NCO: Noncommissioned Officer

NCOIC: Noncommissioned Officer-in-Charge

OIC: Officer-in-Charge

SDK: Skin Decontamination Kit

TAP: Toxicological Agent Protective, e.g., TAP apron

TC: Training Circular

VCL: Vapor Control Line

INDEX

B

C

D

E

F

G

H

I

L

M

N

O

P

R

S

T

U

V

W

PULMONARY AGENTS
CG

SUMMARY

Signs and Symptoms: eye and airway irritation, dyspnea, chest tightness, and **delayed** pulmonary edema.

Detection: **odor** of newly mown hay or freshly cut grass or corn. Neither the M256A1 detector kit nor chemical-agent detector paper (M8 paper, M9 paper) is designed to identify phosgene, but the MINICAMS, Monitox Plus, Draeger tubes, Individual Chemical Agent Detector (ICAD), M18A2, M90, and M93A1 Fox will detect small concentrations of this gas.

Decontamination: **vapor** - fresh air; **liquid** - copious water irrigation.

Management: termination of exposure, ABCs of resuscitation, enforced rest and observation, oxygen with or without positive airway pressure for signs of respiratory distress, other supportive therapy as needed.

CYANIDE
AC, CK

SUMMARY

Signs and Symptoms: few. After exposure to high Ct, seizures, respiratory and cardiac arrest.

Detection: The **M256A1 detector ticket** detects hydrogen cyanide (AC) as vapor or gas in the air, and the M272 kit detects cyanide in water. The ICAD, M18A2, and M90 detectors also detect AC. The CAM, M8A1 automatic chemical agent alarm (ACAA), and M8 and M9 paper do not detect cyanide.

Decontamination: Skin decontamination is usually not necessary because the agents are highly volatile. Wet, contaminated clothing should be removed and the underlying skin decontaminated with water or other standard decontaminants.

Management: ***Antidote:*** intravenous (IV) sodium nitrite and sodium thiosulfate. ***Supportive:*** oxygen, correct acidosis.

MUSTARD
HD, H

SUMMARY

Signs and Symptoms: asymptomatic latent period (hours). Erythema and blisters on the **skin**; irritation, conjunctivitis, corneal opacity, and damage in the **eyes**; mild upper respiratory signs to marked **airway** damage; also gastrointestinal (GI) effects and bone marrow stem cell suppression.

Detection: M256A1, M272 water testing kit, MINICAMS, the ICAD, M18A2, M21 remote sensing alarm, M90, M93A1 Fox, Bubbler, CAM, and DAAMS (but **NOT** the M8A1 automatic chemical agent alarm), M8 paper, or M9 paper.

Decontamination: 0.5% hypochlorite, M291 kit, and water in large amounts.

Management: Decontamination immediately after exposure is the only way to prevent damage. Supportive care of patients - there is no specific therapy.

LEWISITE
L

SUMMARY

Signs and Symptoms: Lewisite causes immediate pain or irritation of skin and mucous membranes. Erythema and blisters on the skin and eye and airway damage similar to those seen after mustard exposures develop later.

Detection: M256A1, M272 water testing kit, MINICAMS, the ICAD, M18A2, M21 remote sensing alarm, M90, M93A1 Fox, Bubbler, CAM, and DAAMS (but **NOT** the M8A1 automatic chemical agent alarm), M8 paper, or M9 paper.

Decontamination: M291, 0.5% hypochlorite, water in large amounts.

Management: immediate decontamination; symptomatic management of lesions the same as for mustard lesions; a specific antidote (BAL) will decrease systemic effects.

PHOSGENE OXIME

CX

SUMMARY

Signs and Symptoms: immediate burning and irritation followed by wheal-like skin lesions and eye and airway damage.

Detection: M256A1, M18A2, M90, and M93 Fox (but **NOT** the M272 water testing kit), MINICAMS, the ICAD, M21 remote sensing alarm, Bubbler, CAM, DAAMS, the M8A1 automatic chemical agent alarm, M8 paper, or M9 paper.

Decontamination: water in large amounts, 0.5% hypochlorite, M291.

Management: immediate decontamination, symptomatic management of lesions.

NERVE AGENTS
GA, GB, GD, GF, VX

SUMMARY

__Signs and Symptoms:__

__Vapor:__

Small exposure -- miosis, rhinorrhea, mild difficulty breathing.

Large exposure -- sudden loss of consciousness, convulsions, apnea, flaccid paralysis, copious secretions, miosis.

__Liquid on skin:__

Small to moderate exposure -- localized sweating, nausea, vomiting, feeling of weakness.

Large exposure -- sudden loss of consciousness, convulsions, apnea, flaccid paralysis, copious secretions.

Detection: M256A1, CAM, M8 paper, M9 paper, M8A1 and M8 alarm systems.

Decontamination: M291, M258A1, hypochlorite, large amounts of water.

Immediate management: administration of MARK I Kits (atropine and pralidoxime chloride); diazepam in addition if casualty is severe; ventilation and suction of airways for respiratory distress.

INCAPACITATING AGENTS
BZ, Agent 15

SUMMARY

Signs and Symptoms: mydriasis; dry mouth; dry skin; increased DTRs; decreased level of concentration; disturbance in perception and interpretation (illusions and/or hallucinations); denial of illness; short attention span; impaired memory.

Detection: No field detector is available.

Decontamination: Gentle, but thorough washing of skin and hair with water or soap and water is required. Bleach is not necessary. Remove clothing.

Management: **Antidote:** physostigmine. **Supportive:** monitoring of vital signs, especially core temperature.

RIOT-CONTROL AGENTS
CS, CN

SUMMARY

Signs and Symptoms: burning and pain on exposed mucous membranes and skin, eye pain and tearing, burning in the nostrils, respiratory discomfort, and tingling of the exposed skin.

Detection: no detector.

Decontamination: **Eyes:** thoroughly flush with water, saline, or similar substance. **Skin:** flush with copious amounts of water, alkaline soap and water, or a mildly alkaline solution (sodium bicarbonate or sodium carbonate). Generally, decontamination is not needed if the wind is brisk. Hypochlorite exacerbates the skin lesion and should not be used.

Immediate management: Usually none is necessary; effects are self-limiting.